Structural Family Therapy

Family Therapy
Theory, Practice, and Technique

Vincent D. Foley, Ph.D. SERIES EDITOR

Private Practice
Bronx, New York

Structural Family Therapy

Carter C. Umbarger, Ph.D.
Director
The Family Institute of Cambridge
Cambridge, Massachusetts

Allyn and Bacon
Boston London Sydney Toronto

A Division of Simon & Schuster
160 Gould Street
Needham Heights, MA 02194

International Standard Book Number 0-205-10169-0

Printed in the United States of America
10 9 8 7 6 5 4 3 2 94 93 92 91 90

For Susan and Jessica,
of course.

CONTENTS

ACKNOWLEDGMENTS

During 1968, while in the midst of a conventional internship at a private, traditionally oriented psychiatric facility outside of Boston, I met Marvin Snider, who first introduced me to family therapy. He supervised the single family case I could find time for and offered the easy-going encouragement that was the only kind possible for someone thoroughly entangled in psychoanalysis, as indeed I was at that time. My research interests, however, were in fact about family matters, and in this I was greatly supported by Drs. Norbett Mintz and Robert A. Rosenthal, both of whom were guiding substantial parts of my work at that time. To pursue these family researches, I made arrangements to join the clinical staff of the Philadelphia Child Guidance Clinic in the fall of 1968.

From 1968 until my return to Boston in 1971 I was a member of the small, consistently exciting clinical and research staff that Salvador Minuchin had been organizing since 1966. The Philadelphia Child Guidance Clinic was really in its golden period, at least for me. The seminars led by Minuchin, the reading groups with Jay Haley, and the daily contact with other beginning family therapists created an atmosphere that was both exhilarating and exhausting. The learning that Minuchin and Haley started in each of us was, luckily for me, grounded in weekly contact with Braulio Montalvo and Neal Daniels, two gifted clinicians and theoreticians who supervised much of my work. It was with them that I learned how to use structural techniques on the daily firing line. One other teacher in the Philadelphia group was especially important to me—the late Rae Weiner, who persisted as an advocate of ideological complexity at a time when most of us were beginning to believe that there was, after all, one right way.

In 1971 Philip Helfaer and Larry Schiff made it possible for me to return to Boston. They helped me establish a family therapy training and clinical program for psychotic adolescents and their families in the Adolescent Service of Boston State Hospital. At the same time, John Pearce, in his generous way, was helping me meet members of the Boston–Cambridge community who had similar interests. He also suggested I write this book. In 1974 I joined with two of these people, David Kantor and Barry Dym, to found The Family Institute of Cambridge. My work and discussions with these two colleagues were enormously helpful in refining some of the ideas that appear here. My personal experience during these early years of the Institute were also immeasurably assisted through the kindly and vital wisdom of Myron Sharaf, who helped me sustain an interest in families without betraying the profound psychologies of individual life.

Barry Dym has given wonderful support and assistance during the months involved in this project and has spent many hours discussing with me all the topics that, were they to have been introduced here, would have made the book quite unmanageable. Several other close friends and colleagues agreed to give the manuscript a critical reading. Sallyann Roth and Richard Chasin, who joined the Institute as directors in 1980, have been wise friends and careful critics, knowing what had to be challenged, what it was possible for me actually to do, and, I have no doubt, knowing what I really could not hear. Caroline Marvin was especially helpful in creating an organizational flow where, prior to her efforts, there was all too often only a confusing maze of ideas. Charles Verge made me reconsider some of the topics addressed in the final chapters and thus made possible a decent ending to things. Richard Bush helped considerably with earlier chapters and, having led the way two years earlier with a book of his own, taught me how to think more carefully about all aspects of writing and publishing. My series editor, Vince Foley, gave a generous amount of time to several careful readings of the manuscript and was calm and considerate throughout the final stages of preparation. Certainly some, if not a good deal, of whatever clarity marks the following pages owes much to the efforts of these friends and readers. Where I have not followed their advice, the consequences are mine to bear or to enjoy, whatever the case.

Susan Conant read and edited all of the first draft. She seldom failed to give me the definitive praises and critiques for which she is justly famous and without which this project would surely have been a less happy venture.

FOREWORD

Family Therapy: Theory, Practice, and Technique began with the concept of producing a whole series of volumes that would explore the spectrum of family therapy for the student or beginning practitioner. As a teacher and supervisor of family therapy for many years, I was aware that there were no books that covered the field adequately. While there were articles and chapters and a few introductions, they all lacked depth. Although there were texts written by some important therapists that did go into more detail, they were beyond the grasp of the beginner. The plan, then, was to produce brief, simple, but comprehensive texts that would cover the field of family therapy broadly and also in depth for those whose actual experience was limited.

The plan developed with three goals. The first was to find authors who were specialists in given areas and who could offer both experience and expertise. The second was to unify the material in a way that would give it continuity so that the different books together would form a coherent whole. The final goal was to stress case material, since experience had shown that students always want to know how theoretical differences translate into practice. Taking the student through the system in a step-by-step manner using clinical examples to illustrate the interplay of theory and practice is the best way to teach exactly how theory can be applied to practice.

For each topic in the series, we asked leaders in the respective fields to suggest the best author. Dr. Umbarger was the overwhelming choice for this first volume, and the text he has written is a justification of that decision. *Structural Family Therapy* is an expert blending of theory, clinical practice, and technique. It strikes exactly the right note as the first volume in the series since it is clear, simple, and heuristic. It is a how-to book in the best sense of the term in that it leads the reader from theory to practice with relevant use of technique.

It is easy to be complex and verbose, and for many, this is impressive. Those of us who teach and supervise, however, realize that it is best to be simple without being simplistic. The real challenge is to compose many various elements in a unified pattern so that a student can make sense of a sometimes overwhelming array of information. Carter Umbarger has done this in *Structural Family Therapy*. I am sure that his text will become the definitive one in the field.

Vincent D. Foley, Ph.D.
Series Editor

PREFACE

This book introduces the major premises of structural family therapy to therapists who, though skilled in other therapeutic modalities, are just beginning their work with families. The present undertaking is oriented to the therapist who requires a basic introduction to general systems theory and a sense of how that theory has been translated into the clinical skills known as structural family therapy. In the chapters that follow I have tried to make an orderly presentation of the theory that underlies the structural approach and then a description of the intervention techniques used by structural therapists. The emphasis here is on the fundamentals of this approach, not on the intricate fine points that may interest the more advanced family therapist. Experienced family clinicians already familiar with the basics of structural family therapy would be well served by Minuchin and Fishman's most recent book, *The Techniques of Family Therapy* (1981).

These basic skills are presented in a way that will, I hope, encourage beginning students to believe that they will eventually master them. Too frequently the power of structural interventions seems more a function of the charm and charisma of the therapist than of the elegant efficiency of the skills themselves. Structural family therapy is a learnable theory of change. It does not require magic, in either therapeutic presence or utterance. Moreover, a good deal of therapy occurs in the muck and mire of the middle phases of effort, not in the dazzle of an unforgettable initial interview. In this spirit I have given attention to what happens after the initial opening with a family and to how one recovers from interventions that fail.

The development of structural family therapy is, of course, authored by Salvador Minuchin and his associates at the Philadelphia Child Guidance Clinic, the best known of whom are Jay Haley (since moved on to work in the "strategic" therapies), Braulio Montalvo, and Harry Aponte. These few have generated a number of important publications that have defined and then elaborated on the meanings of structural therapy. Recent contributions by Minuchin (1981) and Aponte and Van Deusen (1981) appeared after my own efforts to discuss the elements of structural family therapy were well under way. Where possible I have tried to incorporate these recent works when it would not divert the reader's attention from the elemental aspects of structural therapy. At the same time that Minuchin's new work was appearing, important refinements and extensions of systems theory were also being made. I refer to the "second cybernetics" emphasized by Lynn Hoffman (1981) and to the rapid application of these and other systems concepts through the expansion of the "strategic therapies," especially the work of Palazzoli and her associates (1978). The new and compelling uses of the systems paradigm have exciting possibilities, including some useful revisions of the many techniques advised in this book.

The organization of this book is straightforward and, except for the opening chapter on general systems theory, intended to parallel much of the adventure and misadventure one actually experiences when beginning a family case from the structural perspective. Chapters 2, 3, and 4 introduce the beginning therapist to critical issues of joining, data collecting, major terms of the structural orientation, and some presumed advantages of this viewpoint. Chapter 5 tells one how actually to make a structural diagnosis and begin therapy. Chapters 6 and 7 document the major intervention strategies associated with structural therapy. Chapter 8 suggests what happens, and what to do, after all the opening moves are over and brilliant first hopes fade into the menial middle phases of therapy. The final chapter reviews some advantages and problems with this approach and suggests likely directions for those structural therapists who look to the future of their theory.

Structural Family Therapy

Part I

THEORETICAL CONCEPTS

Chapter 1

Character, Context, and Change

The Genogram of Mrs. N.

Consider the following story: Becky, age seven, was referred to therapy by her teacher because of poor adjustments in the classroom. She was often tearful, complaining that she missed her own room at home, and she seemed generally immature in her social behavior. Otherwise she was bright and personable. Her parents accepted the referral since they were concerned about frequent occurrences of similar behavior at home. The parents, both in their mid-30s, brought Becky and her younger brother, age four, to the initial interview. Both parents were college educated, sensitive to emotional issues, and in apparent harmony about their lives. Mrs. N. had previously been in an individual psychotherapy that emphasized family-of-origin issues, complete with intricate genograms of her family tree and periodic "homework" assignments with the surviving members of her family. Mrs. N. considered herself a depressed personality who had greatly benefited from her previous therapy. She was now concerned about her daughter.

During the first half of the interview, Mrs. N. spoke often of her genogram and an apparent "heritage of inadequacy" passed down through her mother's side of the family to the oldest daughters of each generation, a category to which she, her own mother, and now her daughter belonged. Mrs. N. argued, with compelling good sense, that this legacy of social ineptitude was now appearing in Becky. To describe this transmission of inadequacy down through the generations, she used the term "symbiotic transfer," a phrase that carried considerable meaning for her. During Mrs. N.'s efforts to tell her story, the therapist, a young woman, noticed that Becky frequently interrupted her mother, usually by whining or by slumping noisily in her chair. More importantly, the therapist noted that these interruptions seemed part of a simple sequence of behaviors. This sequence was best shown when the mother asked to use the therapist's blackboard to draw her family genogram, at which point the following exchange occurred.

Mother: This whole problem started way back with . . . well, at least my mother's mother. So . . . may I (indicating the blackboard and rising from her chair)? See, the pattern is here (begins to draw a diagram showing several generations of men and women of her extended family) and it's very upsetting . . . and then. . . .

Father: Your mother was . . . well, I think she didn't really expect much of her own mother. (He has interruped his wife as if to help her with the description of her family.) She was really something else! (He turns slightly toward his daughter, sitting opposite him, and whispers) Are you O.K.?

Mother: It really is upsetting to see all this laid out. I just know these women. . . .

Daughter: (Becky leaves her chair and joins mother at the board, picks up a piece of chalk and begins to scribble.) That's stupid. I can't do it (indicating her scribbles). You do it. (She clings to her mother.)

Mother: Becky, don't interrupt. This is mommy's time, then you can have a turn. (She leads Becky firmly back to her seat.) Please let me finish this (said firmly).

Father: (He sits back in his chair, then signals the younger son to come and sit with him. His wife resumes her story.)

In themselves, these brief exchanges among the family members may seem unremarkable, except for their periodic recurrence. The therapist, however, chose to make a rough translation of these behaviors and to convert them into a pattern, which went like this: (1) Mrs. N. would reach back into her past, striving for psychological meaning, but showing some emotional distress as she did so; (2) her husband, in rather neutral tones, would often add some information, but then invariably interact with his daughter, usually checking to see if she was "O.K."; (3) Becky, after such contact, would generally begin interrupting her mother, who (4) would respond quite competently and return her daughter to her seat, (5) at which point the husband relaxed his vigilance. When this sequence next began to appear, the therapist decided to intervene. Table 1-1 presents the two ways she could so this.

The structural intervention shown in Table 1-1 attends to the father's role in the behavioral exchange and indirectly addresses the way he cues his daughter to worry that someone (probably his wife) might not be "O.K." The therapist's remark accommodates to this preference for indirect communication; she does not ask Mrs. N. to reassure her husband directly,

Table 1-1
POSSIBLE THERAPIST INTERVENTIONS IN THE PROBLEM OF MRS. N.'S DAUGHTER

Problem	Structural Intervention	Alternative Intervention
How to stop the daughter from interrupting and clinging to her mother.	"Mrs. N., would you tell your husband to remind Becky that you are fine, that this is an old story of yours, and you don't need any help with it. That you know exactly what to do. Ask your husband to do that for you."	"It would be good to stop her from that because, see, she is identifying with you, acting inadequate right now, just like you feel yourself. So, she wants to be like you, to cling to inadequacy."

but instead to reassure him through the child and to involve him as a competent parent who is himself capable of reassuring the daughter that her mother is "O.K." At some later point, one might wish to encourage a more direct exchange between the parents, leaving the daughter out.

Table 1-1 also shows an alternative intervention, which has merit from a psychodynamic perspective and correctly addresses issues of learned role behavior or identification. This intervention does not, however, interrupt the sequence of behaviors that keep joining mother and daughter together over issues of inadequacy, nor does it alter the father's rather peripheral position. In symbolic terms, the two interventions have the following structural impact:

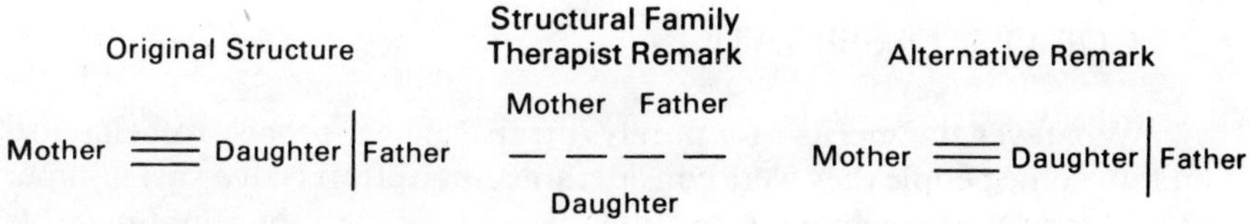

The alternative intervention, however correct with regard to psychological constructs, such as the process of identification, does not change the family organization. The structural intervention does achieve such a rearrangement, bringing the parents together in an hierarchical union that disrupts the enmeshment between Mrs. N. and her daughter.

Structural interventions, once developed, seem sensible and compelling, particularly if one knows when in the therapeutic process they may have the greatest impact. Yet it is not easy to understand or apply these strategies unless one undergoes a change-of-mind about why people act as they do. Therapists interested in learning the techniques of structural family therapy need to understand that it is based on a theory of human behavior that shares little with the psychodynamic paradigm, which for 50 years has governed most therapeutic procedures. That paradigm—more mechanistic in its arrangements of one's interior life and quite linear in its assumptions about causality—seemed, for some time, to guide therapists sufficiently in their efforts to heal behavioral disturbances. But an increasing number of curious observations about people in treatment began, in the 1950s, to interest clinicians in alternative views of human activity. These observations coincided with a rising interest in the natural sciences in a new paradigm of causality, that of the organismic whole, as embodied in the principles of *general systems theory*.

In this paradigm, causality is circular, and behavior has as much to do with one's interactional context as one's interior mental processes. Structural family therapy is one pragmatic derivative from this organismic paradigm, and as developed by Minuchin (1974) and his colleagues, thus far represents the best psychotherapeutic expression of the general systems view of behavior. While in the final chapter more will be said about the contrasts between the mechanistic and the organismic paradigms, the immediate task is to discuss those observations that prompted interest in a new model of behavior and to achieve at least an introductory familiarity with the basic terms of general systems theory. Without such introductions, however formal and brief, the reader will find it difficult to understand how a structural intervention freed Mrs. N. from the tangles of her psychological genogram.

CURIOUS OBSERVATIONS

Whatever the merits of a purely intrapsychic approach to behavior, and for some people they were considerable, such efforts left a vast number of problems both unchanged and unexplained. For example, innumerable clinical reports emerged, especially regarding children, which suggested that a person who behaved well in one setting, e.g., in the therapist's office, behaved very badly elsewhere, e.g., at home. In particular, child guidance workers noted the persistence with which progress in individual child therapy seemed seriously slowed, even reversed, when the child reentered the family. Although this was not invariably so, the instability of change apparently associated with living in the family context could not be ignored. Similar observations were made of anorectic patients: they frequently improved a good deal in the hospital, but reversed this change and regressed when they returned to the family. Another observation difficult to reconcile with the analytic paradigm was the *sequential* appearance of several symptomatic children within the same family. If the improvement in one child held, then a second child would shortly appear symptomatic, although generally each child's symptom differed from the other's. Haley (1963) made a similar observation in his treatment of couples: he might effectively treat the symptoms of one spouse only to be confronted, a short time thereafter, by the other spouse, now also symptomatic.

Even more unsettling were the events observed by Bateson, Jackson, Haley, and Weakland (1956) in their studies of schizophrenic adults. Whatever the individual interior pathology, there were severe and disturbing alterations in the patient's language and other behaviors when interviewed with other family members. Attention to the patient's historical troubles seemed less compelling than the contemporary disturbances enacted when patient and family met together. All of these observations, which were difficult to reconcile with the prevailing model of change, pointed to a new source of influence—namely, that of the interactional context over its individual members.

FROM CHARACTER TO CONTEXT

The shift from exclusive concerns with individual character to a focus on interactional context was enormously facilitated by the development of the general systems theory paradigm. Although the initial impetus for a revolution in paradigms came from biology, cybernetics, and information theory, the behavioral sciences soon saw that some of the "curious observations" just noted might be better understood through a model that emphasized circular, rather than linear, causality. This is exactly what the "systems" or "organismic" paradigm did emphasize, along with a variety of other new, key concepts about the interrelatedness of individuals to their behavioral context. The emphasis on wholism, on the organic integrity and complexity of any living entity, also implied a *systematic* organization of this complexity. Thus, the interdependent parts of any living entity were organized into relational patterns, which were themselves larger and different in meaning than a simple summing-up of the parts. Each system so organized was characterized by certain rules and operational routines that defined how the subordinate parts related to each other and how they in turn influenced the purpose of the larger system. From this systems paradigm of human activity were derived the theoretical terms of structural family therapy.

The remainder of this chapter presents a brief introduction to the principal features of the general systems paradigm. Chapter 2 will discuss how these abstractions are turned into the concrete terms of structural theory and therapy.

PRINCIPAL FEATURES OF THE SYSTEMS PARADIGM

A System

A system is a set of units, organized and interdependent, standing in interactional relation to each other. It is a set of interrelated elements with a capacity for performance, especially in regard to adaptation to the surrounding environment. Two points are important for our discussion. First, a system—whether a single cell, an organ, a body, or a family group—is, in this discussion, always a *living* system. As such, it exists in a state of perpetual exchange with the environment around it. This exchange activity *is* the context within which life is organized, develops, changes, and finally dies. For families, the context of exchange includes their social class, their ethnicity, the surrounding culture of their particular geographical setting, and even their time in universal history. Second, the frequent reference to the "parts" of a system and to their interrelatedness means that any system is composed of *subsystems* or *subunits* (interchangeable terms), which are themselves both servants and architects of the rules and routines that make up the organized whole. These subunits stand in dynamic relationship to each other and are organized around the performance of functions crucial to the survival of the total system.

A Boundary

A boundary may be experienced as rule-governed transactions that regularly occur between people over long periods of time. For units smaller than a social group, such as a cell or organ, the boundary may be palpable as, for example, the skin of our bodies. But in family groups, the boundary is an interactive phenomenon occurring over time. Such boundaries help achieve and define the separateness between the subunits of the total system. In families, boundary properties may vary according to the subunit involved and the adaptive task being undertaken. The easiest way to understand boundaries within family units is to examine the verbal and nonverbal behaviors that both allow and prohibit the transfer of information about life. For example, parents may routinely, throughout time, prohibit their children from knowing certain things about their marriage. This censorship of information creates a tight boundary around the marital subunit. Conversely, the whole family unit may routinely, throughout time, allow and invite many different types of friends and interests to become part of the family's life. This is an open-family-unit boundary (see Fig. 1-1).

Without boundaries, a variety of critical family process developments will not occur; there can be no progressive differentiation of functions in the individuals or in the separate subunits, and hence no systems complexity. Without systems complexity, there is a drastically reduced ability to create and maintain an adaptive stance *vis-à-vis* the surrounding environment. Without adaptation, the system is in trouble, its individual parts begin to show symptomatic strain, and the forces of entropy and decay soon prevail.

But what do boundaries keep in and let out? What do they regulate? Boundaries regulate the flow of information and energy required by a living system in its constant business of maintaining harmonious balance with its environmental context. Indeed, the concepts of information and of energy are central to a general systems theory of family process; they form the basic stuff of a family's daily activity. *Information* refers to verbal and nonverbal signals that tell how well any part of the system, or the system as a whole, is measuring up to some ideal goals or purposes. If, for example, parents believe that they should be the ones to convey all sexual information to their children, then they will signal disapproval when a child brings home a sex education manual from school. *Energy,* a more elusive phenomenon, refers to the emotional force, repetition, and duration of any particular signal. Using the above example, the parents may become angry and punishing, reminding the child of the rule against bringing such reading material into the family. Or the parents may

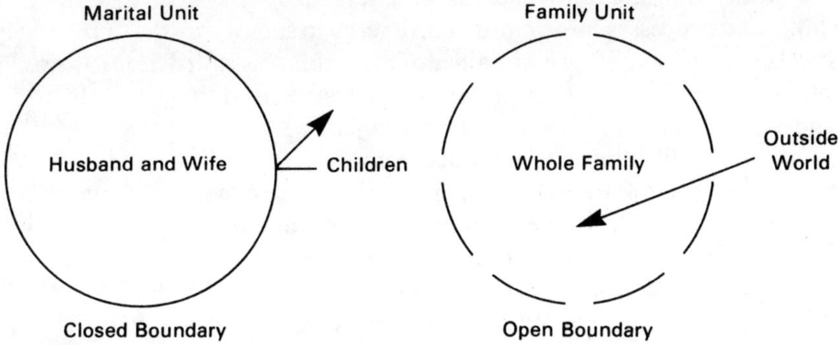

FIGURE 1-1. A closed boundary around the marital subunit (left) and an open-family-unit boundary (right).

mention the issue only once, soon forget about it, and even, at a later time, prove inconsistent on this point. Energy refers to the force and the rate of exchange evident around the transmission of these information signals.

Feedback and System Design

Inputs and outputs of information and energy are conveyed through a cybernetic event designated as a *feedback loop*. For families, feedback loops are communicational pathways that circle across unit boundaries and back again, signaling to the members of that unit their degree of conformity or difference from the overall purpose of the system. All systems are "about something"; that is, they are all in some state of more or less adaptive exchanges with the environment. The *design* of a system refers to the goal of these exchanges and the style in which exchanges are made. Families arrive at these superordinate designs for living in a variety of ways. Structural family theorists have given little attention to a typology of family process, though others have attempted a variety of classificatory schemes (Beavers, 1977; Kantor & Lehr, 1975). Regardless of the characteristic way in which any one family proceeds to create the design for an adaptive living-in-context, it must be disseminated throughout the entire family group, conveyed accurately to each subunit, which in turn must process and respond to that information. Thus, there is a constant flow and exchange of information and energy across the boundaries of the interdependent parts. This flow is chiefly organized through two types of feedback loops: those loops that promote stability or homeostasis in the system and those loops that promote growth and change.

Feedback and Homeostasis

Many times, adaptiveness is best served by a system that remains stable and processes information and energy in such a way that a relatively steady state of activity is maintained. This stability is called *homeostasis* or *systems equilibrium* and is necessary for a system to function effectively and without undue stress on its component parts. Feedback loops that promote equilibrium may be called *constancy loops*, indicating that the function of feedback activity is to maintain a state of constancy or relative sameness in how the family goes about its business. More formally, these feedback loops are called *deviation-countering loops*. Simply put, one discovers some behavioral baseline or norm and notes that deviations from this norm are "countered"; that is, they evoke a family reaction that brings the behavior back to the previous baseline. When the behavior is successfully countered, then it must either be abandoned entirely or altered so that it has a close enough fit with the prevailing systems design. The following is an example of a deviation-countering feedback loop that promotes homeostasis.

During the interview of a family with a highly disturbed adolescent girl (diagnosed as psychotic), the therapist noticed that the parents always spoke clearly and rationally while their daughter, Sara, always mumbled and seemed irrational. In order to test this observation and to determine whether a baseline behavior was present, the therapist created an opportunity for a different behavior to occur.

Therapist: Now I would like to hear from Sara, from her only. What did happen before the police came?
Daughter: It was 6:30, and I was listening to the radio in my room. . . . (She begins to give a clear and audible account of events.)
Mother: (Raises her hand to her mouth, covers it briefly.)
Father: (Raises his hand to his mouth, covers it briefly.)
Daughter: I think I've said enough for now. . . . I don't really remember anymore.

The parents successfully signaled their daughter that she had strayed an unacceptable distance from a baseline expectation. They silently covered their mouths, and Sara stopped speaking. She became silent and slightly confused and was now in compliance with a family norm. Homeostasis was restored. Although in this example, the successful countering of the daughter's new move seemed to restore an unhappy equilibrium, there was nothing inherently wrong with homeostatic states as long as they could also yield to periods of growth and change.

Feedback and Growth

The notion of a homeostatic state is only half the story about family life. Any living system must always be in a state of dynamic tension, alternating between pressures for growth and further differentiation, and states of periodic rest and stasis, those momentary plateaus that provide some respite and relief from the pains of growing. The emphasis on a system's capacity for growth and change is surprisingly new. Early students of family process were most impressed by a family's capacity to "return to normal" (whatever that might mean for them), that is, by the capacity for homeostatic control. Now, theorists like Maruyama (1968), Hoffman (1981), and Dell (1981, 1982) have emphasized the equally essential, though perhaps less observable, ability for systems to grow and to transform their very essence in order to accommodate to the needs of individual members as well as the pressures of the changing environment. The feedback loops that promote growth may be called *variety loops,* indicating that the outcome of the feedback activity is to sanction diversity and difference, thereby creating new behavioral baselines. More formally, these feedback loops are called *deviation-amplifying loops.* As opposed to deviation-countering loops, which promote constancy and unity of purpose, the deviation-amplifying loop promotes growth and diversity. When some new behavioral event or sequence occurs, it evokes reinforcing responses from other family members that ensure the survival of the new behavior. The following is an example of a deviation-amplifying feedback loop that promotes growth.

A mother and father seemed in total, though despairing, agreement that their two latency-age children, Karen and Tony, were mean and unmanageable. The mother was especially angry at Karen, claiming that the daughter hated her and deliberately irritated her. While the parents talked with the therapist, both children continually left their seats and ran in circles around both parents, constantly reaching out to touch them as they passed by. Finally, the father reached out, gathered up Tony, and sat him firmly on his lap. The son quieted down. But the mother continued her angry comments about Karen, noting that they hated to touch each other and were never affectionate with each other. The therapist then initiated the following sequence.

Therapist: (Speaking to mother) I wonder if you couldn't hold your daughter on your lap, like your husband is doing with Tony.

Mother: Oh no. Karen wouldn't have any of that. She *hates* being touched. Besides, I don't feel comfortable in that stuff.

Father: (Speaking to his wife) You should do it . . . go on . . . try. Karen, go over to your mother.

Daughter: (Moves toward the mother and sits on her lap.)

Father: (Speaking to his wife) You are doing good. That's good like that.

Therapist: I notice Karen seems more relaxed. She's smiling.

Mother: (Begins to cry, her body softens) This is silly, but she's not so bad.

The new behavior, affectionate physical contact between mother and daughter, was reinforced in several ways: first, the father encouraged his wife to accept the therapist's suggestion, then the daughter showed visible pleasure, and finally, the mother amplified her own new behavior through her tears and a softening of her anger. Growth and change in this area will be helpful for the family before it reaches another plateau of homeostatic rest.

The conceptual advantages of a general systems approach to family process can be appreciated in these notions of homeostasis and growth, for they are basically a way of understanding family unity and individual diversity and of attending to the inescapable reality that while all life forms must change, they must also maintain enough regularity and balance to continue an adaptive interchange with the surrounding environmental context. The living unit must grow, but in a way, it must also stay the same. Change and growth will occur, but in a manner and at a rate that preserves a sense of sameness. A healthy family, from this viewpoint, appears charmingly conservative, seeming to remain the same while nonetheless subtly promoting growth and change within its individual subunits.

Structure

The term *structure* refers to relatively enduring interactional patterns that serve to arrange or organize a family's component subunits into somewhat constant relationships. These patterned alliances and coalitions among family members are the structures that regulate a family's daily flow of information and energy. In this sense, a structure is not a static container of an interpersonal exchange, but a metaphor for regularly occurring behavioral exchanges. As Minuchin has put it, a structure refers to ". . . the invisible set of functional demands that organizes the ways in which family members interact" (1974, p. 51). These definitions emphasize a dynamic attribute of structures—that of the active organization of behavior into predictable routines. But the more popular connotation of structure is that of something still or static, of something fixed in time, as though one might suddenly freeze the family's interactive life and thereby create a "structure." This connotation points to an important distinction—that between structure and process.

Structure and Process

A process refers to a discrete, time-limited sequence of behaviors that make up any particular transaction. A family decision process, for example, may be observed to consist of several linked behaviors: the father makes some opening statement, his oldest son opposes him, and the mother comes to the support of her son, this mother–son arrangement having enough force to determine an outcome. When a temporal dimension is added, a distinction may be made between structure and process. The expression of a process over time gives that process the status of a structure. If, in the example, the mother and son *repeatedly,* over time, join forces against the father's effort to direct a decision, then one may speak of a mother–son *coalitional structure.* Where such an arrangement does not persist over time, then the observer has simply witnessed a brief, transitional process in the evolving movement of family life and not an enduring structure.

Using the temporal term "duration" to make the same point, von Bertalanffy has noted that ". . . structures are slow processes of long duration" (1968, p. 27). One may also imagine the converse, that processes are structural arrangements of very short duration. Imagine the animated comic books of children. Here is an arrangement of hundreds of "structures," the pages, each one a static drawing arrived at by an invariant movement of the pen, thereby ensuring a recognizable form rather than a random scribble. This "structure," the drawing, is the result of artistic constancy over time. Yet under the pressure of an energetic thumb, these hundreds of pages can become "structures of short duration," creating an animated and usually amusing story (in this case, the "process" of the narrative). But if the thumb is raised, the rapid interactional process stops, and one is once again confronted with a "structure," a static line drawing, perhaps of Donald Duck. Structure and process may then, in part, be defined in terms of the other by adding the temporal notion of duration.

Structure and Content

Although structural family therapy often seems to ignore the psychological content that is the focus of the analytic paradigm, general systems theory provides some perspective on this matter. *Content* refers to the particular themes and concretized attributes of life, which, strung together, give thematic substance to the concepts of information and energy. The hopes, dreams, envies, loves, memories, and aspirations of people's daily lives make up the content of individual phenomenal experience. But what is the relation of this content to a systems view of family structure and process?

Very simply, one may select for study any content theme, such as personal identity images, family ideals, or parental power, or one may postulate that human activity is about anything, such as the defense against forbidden impulses, the organization of mental operations into automatic response patterns, and so forth. But once the content theme has been selected, one needs to recognize that it, per se, is only of secondary importance, at least from a systems perspective. Primarily, general systems theory (1) recognizes and examines the structures created by the transactional expression of content; and (2) emphasizes the behavioral operations whereby any discrete item of content makes its way across a boundary and, transformed by the very act of boundary crossing, then impacts on the surrounding interpersonal environment. What goes on inside a bounded unit are the events often designated *content*, but such events become observable, and hence available for a systems analysis, only when they make up a *behavior-exchange sequence* occurring across unit boundaries. (See Fig. 1-2.)

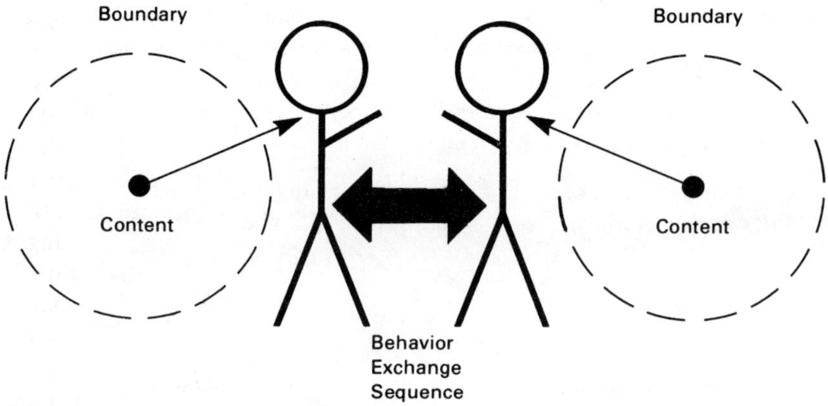

FIGURE 1-2. Behavior-exchange sequence occurring across unit boundaries. Content—events going on within the bounded unit—is observable only when it occurs across unit boundaries and becomes available for a systems analysis.

These sequences are largely informational and energetic in nature and consequently comprise exactly the right data for a general systems analysis of family procedures. The content studied is of secondary interest; how it is transformed through a series of behavior-exchange sequences in such a way as to remain congruent with the family's design for living becomes the proper focus of a systems analysis.

Seeing Structure

Seeing structure is at first difficult. It sounds abstract, and it requires one to overlook interesting matters of content, the psychological nuts and bolts that traditionally command therapeutic attention. Actually, one can learn to spot structures by attending to the more elemental aspects of behavioral exchanges rather than to the intricacies of meaning that burden most communications. Here is an example of seeing structure.

The Conrad family sought help because Mrs. Conrad was continually angry at their 11-year-old son, an only child, who she felt was disrespectful, rebellious, and potentially delinquent, and who had struck her on several occasions. Both she and her husband were in their mid-30s and worked in professional capacities. Mr. Conrad came because his wife was so upset. During the initial interview, the father and son exchanged frequent glances and made side remarks to each other. This was particularly evident whenever Mrs. Conrad tried to tell the therapist about her many concerns. The father, when invited by the therapist to give his viewpoint, offered only mild support for his wife and soon fell silent. Efforts to have him discuss matters with his wife also quickly withered. Whenever Mrs. Conrad spoke directly to either her husband or son, they responded very briefly or not at all.

Given this behavior, here are the structures that can be "seen" in the Conrad family:

1. The continual verbal and nonverbal exchange between father and son *is a structure*, in this case an enmeshed alliance.

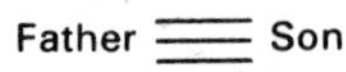

2. The persistently weak response given by the husband to the wife *is a structure,* in this case a diffuse/weak alliance.

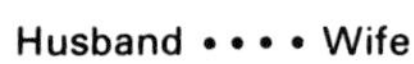

3. The constant deflection of the mother's remarks by the husband and son *is a structure,* in this case a closely bounded dyad that actually excludes the mother.

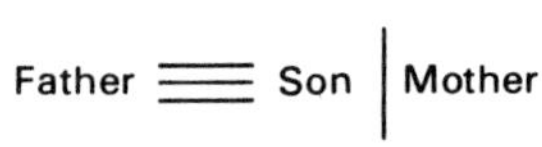

4. On the basis of these observed structures, the therapist might infer that the father–son dyad is actually a cross-generational coalition against the mother. This *is a structural hypothesis.*

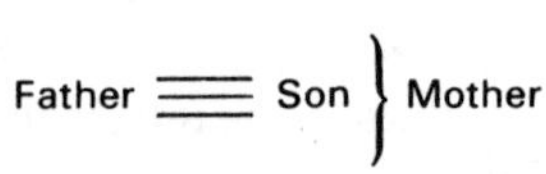

These are the structures that can be "seen" and are representative of the observations that comprise the data of a structural diagnosis.

SUMMING UP THE SYSTEMS PARADIGM

The case for a general systems model of behavior is not being argued here nor extensively presented. Readers interested in a fuller elaboration of these ideas can turn to the works of von Bertalanffy (1968), Buckley (1967), Miller (1965), or the easier-to-grasp writings of Hoffman (1981) or

Walrond-Skinner (1976). Although only briefly presented, the systems paradigm of behavior underlies all major propositions of structural family therapy and so requires at least this initial attention before moving to the therapeutic procedures derived from it. For therapists, the most important features of this paradigm are the following:

1. *Part and whole.* It is not the individual part or isolated content that deserves initial attention, but the larger system (itself greater and different than simply the sum of its parts) and the transactional process within this system. This system *is* the environmental context in which any part functions and in which any particular content occurs.
2. *Information, error, and feedback.* Living systems have communication-feedback loops that give information about the activities of the system. This information consists of "error" signals that tell any given subunit whether or not its behavior is dissimilar to the overall design for living of the total system.
3. *Feedback and homeostasis.* When information signals a difference from some baseline of the overall design, deviation-countering behaviors may occur. They induce constancy of homeostasis in the system, a steady state of being that is necessary for life.
4. *Feedback and growth.* When information signals a difference from some baseline of the overall design, deviation-amplifying behaviors may occur. They induce change and diversity in the system, a fluctuating state of being that is necessary for life.
5. *Life and tension.* The continual alteration of periods of growth with periods of stability (of morphogenesis with morphostasis) makes up the dynamic tension of life.
6. *Circularity.* Cause and effect are now viewed as circular, not as linear.
7. *Change.* Change in the total system as well as in any individual part occurs with intervention into the whole as well as into any part. Both part and whole must change in some conjunction with each other, though not always simultaneously.

CHANGE IN CONTEXT

The context within which any particular biological or psychological event occurs refers to all of the properties of a living system just summarized. A context exists (1) when there is a collectivity of parts that surround and stand in an adjacent and dynamic relationship to any particular focal component; and (2) when the transactions that occur among the parts conform to the principles of general systems theory.

The implications for therapeutic change are vastly different when the therapist considers the whole instead of the part, the surrounding context instead of the isolated event, and the family instead of the person. Both clinicians and researchers, using this new paradigm, may now refocus their attention, moving away from the sometimes imponderable constructs of inner life to more observable behaviors in the here and now. It is a move, as Rabkin (1970) would call it, from inner to outer space, from 50 years of preoccupation with what is assumed to go on inside the mind to an increasingly careful observation of what people actually do to and with each other when meeting in the world around them. Students of human behavior have begun to take seriously what good ethologists have known all along—that the animal must be studied in its natural environmental surroundings and that even the most biologically instinctual behaviors become emergent and organizing forces only in relationship to some larger, superordinate context.

Minuchin has put it simply: "When the structure of the family group is transformed, the positions of members in that group are altered accordingly. As a result, each individual's experiences change" (1974, p. 2). That is the basic, though often understated, presumption of a therapy based on systems theory: if the structural context is altered, so will the individual character change. This position reverses the assumptions of the psychoanalytic paradigm, that the individual character is the proper site of therapeutic change. Now it is the context that must be changed, then follow differences in individual behavior.

This conception of change is one way in which structural family therapists elaborate the concepts of systems theory into a model for therapeutic intervention. In the next chapter other elaborations are described so that one may quickly have the fundamental terms of structural therapy.

Chapter 2

The Terms of Structural Family Therapy

Structural family therapy converts the abstractions of general systems theory into descriptions of routine family life and into prescriptions for therapeutic intervention. In this chapter, the major theoretical terms and perspectives of the structural approach are introduced through a focus on normal family development, family pathology, and family therapy. The terms and viewpoints of a systems and structural approach are, as the reader by now knows, usually unfamiliar and difficult to grasp. To speak in systems and structural language is generally like speaking in a foreign tongue. But as in learning any foreign language, it seems helpful to speak only that language while actively learning it. That advice is followed here. There will be little reference to the familiar language and terms of individual psychology, but instead a consistent use of a systems vocabulary to describe the ordinary phenomena of family living. Even partial mastery of this chapter, and the one before it, will give one enough fluency to do more than simply ask directions to the bathroom or bar. We begin by seeing how the structuralists look at normal family development.

A SYSTEMS VIEW OF NORMAL FAMILY DEVELOPMENT

Minuchin wrote in 1974 that ". . . an effectively functioning family is an open social system in transformation, maintaining links with the extrafamilial, possessing a capacity for development, and having an organizational structure composed of subsystems" (p.255). By 1981, he and Fishman had extended this notion to include the more elaborated statement of Prigogine (Glansdorff & Prigogine, 1971)—namely, that living systems are composed of "dissipative structures," that is, of structures that are not simply in a permanent steady state, as are the structures of a crystal. The structures of a living system must always be in some state of flux and *in this way* able to achieve new orders of complexity and new levels of adaptive organization. Old structures dissipate and, in the flux of their dissipation, are replaced by new ones that, in their turn and in their time, under the evolutionary demands of the surrounding environment, will also disappear. Minuchin and Fishman wrote: "In a living system, fluctuations, occurring either internally or externally, take the system to a new structure . . ." (1981, p.21). They then continued, quoting Prigogine:

> . . .[A] new structure is always the result of an instability. It originates from a fluctuation. Whereas a fluctuation is normally followed by a response that brings the system back to the unperturbed state, [as in closed systems] . . . on the contrary, at the point of formation of a new structure, fluctuations are amplified (p.21).

They noted, as have other recent theorists, that the field of family therapy has for too long emphasized the ability of family systems to maintain themselves. A theory of family development needs to emphasize equally a system's ability to transform itself, reaching new states of complexity and adaptive differentiation of structure.

To discuss the evolution of a family system, Minuchin and Fishman, following Koestler (1979), introduced the term *holon* to describe entities that are simultaneously a whole unto themselves and a part of some other, superordinate whole. Koestler's term is based on the Greek *holos* (whole) with the suffix *on*, suggesting a particle or part, as in prot*on*. The term *holon* can then be used to describe large collectivities, like the sibling holon, two person units, like a mother and child holon (thereby escaping such pathognomic words as *symbiosis*), and even the individual holon.

Minuchin and Fishman used this term throughout their 1981 study, because for a therapist, ". . . the unit for intervention is always a holon" (p.13). They described attributes of the holon:

> Every holon—the individual, the nuclear family, the extended family, and the community—is both a whole and a part, not more one than the other, not one rejecting or conflicting with the other. A holon exerts competitive energy for autonomy and self-preservation as a whole. It also carries integrative energy as a part. The nuclear family is a holon of the extended family, the extended family of the community, and so on. Each whole contains the part, and each part also contains the "program" that the whole imposes. Part and whole contain each other in a continuing, current, and ongoing process of communication and interrelationship (p.13).

The individual as a separate subsystem, or holon, developing in context, has been given considerable attention by Minuchin. As he wrote in 1974, "The old idea of the individual acting upon his environment has here become the concept of the individual interacting with his environment . . . a man is not himself without his circumstances" (p.5). He objected to those views of the individual self that have suggested that the family context is actually inimical to personal development, that one needs to be completely "differentiated" from one's family as a measure of true emotional health. On the contrary, a human being must be seen as existing primarily in an interpersonal context. Just as there are no true hermits (but only persons who exist through perpetual and imaginary dialogue with those people they shun), the structural perspective argues that individual identity and individual "mind" exist only as constructs of the interpersonal context. There is no opposition to strictly interior attributes of individuality, such as genetic features; but, in balance, personal identity is believed to develop primarily in interaction with the interpersonal context. "The individual holon incorporates the concept of self-in-context. It includes the personal and historical determinants of self. But it goes beyond them to include the current input of the social context" (Minuchin & Fishman, 1981, p.14). Following Bateson (1972), structuralists have argued that the most prominent characteristics of the individual, including the notion of "mind," are those determined by membership in a human group, originally and most powerfully, the family. As Minuchin argued, ". . . an individual's psychic life is not entirely an internal process. The individual influences his context and is influenced by it in constantly recurring sequences of interaction. . . . His actions are governed by the characteristics of the system . . ." (1974, p.9).

There are three important points here. First, this model gives individual activity the power to alter the surrounding context. This is in accordance with a truly cybernetic model, though often proponents of structural family therapy have been reluctant to give much attention to the individual as such for fear it would involve them with matters of intrapsychic psychology. Structuralism, at least theoretically, gives the individual a place in the cybernetic loop. Second, the passage just cited from Minuchin's 1974 work shows a total compatibility to a general systems view of behavior: that an individual is continually involved in reciprocities with the environment, each influencing the other through a circular model of cause and effect. This is not a new position in the behavioral sciences, but the structuralists have made it more emphatic than others have through the persistent reevaluation of individual psychology as bound to the interpersonal context. The special theoretical contribution of this model is to return consistently to these interactional structures, showing how they constrain and shape the individuals within the system. Third, there is an important corollary to be added: that the interior experience of an individual changes as the context in which he or she lives changes. The notion that an altered context leads to an altered individual character is an axiom of structural family therapy that contrasts sharply with models of change in other schools of psychotherapy.

The development of self-in-context and, alternatively, the modification of context-around-self are the major themes of a structural view of normal family development. This is the task of life: to blend the diversity of individual growth with the unity of family group membership. The varieties of personal, self-actualizing behavior must also balance with the constancies of the total system as it spins through time, adjusting to the continually changing demands of its own environmental context. "The family is an open system in transformation; that is, it constantly receives and sends inputs to and from the extrafamilial, and it adapts to the different demands of the developmental stages it faces" (Minuchin, 1974, p.50). Moreover, this process of individual socialization and family development is basically conflictual; hence the necessity for always finding a balance, a norm that preserves both the individual and the system. Within the family system, transactional patterns develop to ensure that the behavior of individual members will be regulated in accordance with the larger agenda, that of the family's survival in the surrounding world. These patterns are maintained by two sources of constraint. The first is generic and involves the universal rules governing family organization. For example, some form of power hierarchies and role complementarity is required in all forms of social organization. The second source of constraint is idiosyncratic, the highly personalized configuration given, over the years, by a family to the various daily routines it carries out through the course of its life. Explicit in these formulations, and in much of Minuchin's discussion of pathology is a concept of the family life cycle, beginning with the couple's marriage and ending with their return to primary spouse roles after the children have grown.

To describe more completely how the normal family develops into a viable system, serving both itself and the more discrete needs of its subunits, structuralists have noted three major features of a family group.

First, the family group is divided into subsystems, often arranged in hierarchical positions, sometimes by definition, as in parents and children, and sometimes by functional reality, as in divisions between obedient sibs and the rebellious sibs. Minuchin (1974) gave these subsystems considerable prominence in his view of family development: "The subsystem organization . . . provides valuable training in the process of maintaining the differentiated 'I am' while exercising interpersonal skills at different levels" (p.53). Individuals belong to different subsystems and, in these varying contexts, learn different skills for living.

Second, subsystems are created and endure through the establishment of clear boundaries that routinely separate and protect their specialized functions from those of other subsystems. Actually, the concept of boundary is too often given a concreteness that isolates it from the living processes of daily behavior. A boundary is not a magic-marker line on some clinician's diagram of the family's structure. A boundary is a metaphor about accessibility to a holon. This metaphor shows the way and the rules for how one enters into contact with various units of the family system. The particular metaphorical qualities of any given boundary (e.g., whether it is described as open or closed) depend exclusively on the routine behavioral transactions that, *over time*, consistently regulate the flow of informational and energetic traffic from one holon to another.

The metaphor of boundaries is defined very like the metaphor of structure—both are constructs that refer to *recurring* behavioral exchanges between the members of adjacent holons. In one sense, boundaries are the occasion for a structure to exist. Without permanent boundary activity, no structure would form; there would be only endless sequences of new behaviors. Fortunately there is a good deal of redundancy in family life, however. Boundaries emerge, and structures do form. Clearly, then, the function of boundaries is to protect the differentiation of the system and to allow for the emergence of structure.

There is, in summary, no adaptive, open family system that does not differentiate itself into holons or subsystems. These holons come about through the development of both generic and idiosyncratic behavioral transactions. The repetition of these transactions ensures the durability and viability of the subsystem. The metaphors of boundary and structure are used to describe the arrangement of these subsystems *vis-à-vis* each other and the degree of contact between them. The durabilities of any subsystems are relative, however, and must alternate with the need of the entire system to continue a pattern of dissipative structures and their replacement by new and more complex ones. In this way, "normal family development includes fluctuation, periods of crisis, and resolution at a higher level of complexity" (Minuchin & Fishman, 1981, p.27).

A SYSTEMS VIEW OF FAMILY PATHOLOGY

As already noted about normal development:

> . . . [A] family is subject to inner pressure coming from developmental changes in its own members and subsystems and to outer pressure coming

> from demands to accommodate to the significant social institutions that have an impact on family members. Responding to these demands from both within and without requires a constant transformation of the position of family members in relation to one another, so they can grow while the family system maintains continuity (Minuchin, 1974, p.60).

It follows that pathology connotes a marked and persistent failure to negotiate these stresses in a reasonable way. "The label of pathology would be reserved for families who in the face of stress increase the *rigidity of their transactional patterns* and boundaries, and avoid or resist any exploration of alternatives" (Minuchin, 1974, p.60). When a family operates normally it adapts to the inevitable stresses of life in a way that preserves family continuity while facilitating restructuring. When, however, a family reacts to stress with rigidity, dysfunctional behaviors occur. This is family pathology, and its site is in the family group as a whole, not in an individual member.

Consistent with a general systems view that normal family development requires alterations of homeostasis with periods of crisis and fluctuation, Minuchin and Fishman have noted that a family ". . . is in difficulty because it is stuck in the homeostatic phase . . ." (1981, p.26). Ironically, it is the *absence of a system crisis* that characterizes a family immobilized by the homeostatic machinery of a developmental phase made increasingly obsolete by the requirements for change that come either from within the family group or from the larger environmental surrounding.

Throughout the many case examples described by structuralists, one discerns four major categories of family pathology: pathologies of boundary, alliance, triangle, and hierarchy. Each is naturally a partial culprit in the other categories. Thus, for example, it is difficult to have a pathology of alliances without simultaneously confronting a pathology of boundaries. Nonetheless, the categories are useful for summarizing a structural view of pathology.

Pathology of Boundaries

Family subsystems are less notable for their membership than for the quality of their boundaries. A parental subsystem, for example, may beneficially be composed of a mother and a grandmother, or a mother and a parental child. Trouble arises only when the boundary behaviors of those subsystem participants become inappropriately rigid or weak, thereby impeding an adaptive transmission of information to and from the surrounding subsystems. The version of boundary pathology offered by

Minuchin (1974) can be anchored in systems theory. He argued for a boundary dimension ranging from disengaged to enmeshed and encompassing a normal range.

The enmeshed family system is characterized by the extreme sensitivity of its individual members to each other and to their primary subsystem. There is often little interpersonal distance, considerable blurring of subsystem boundaries, and inappropriately rapid and forceful responses to the activity of family members. "The behavior of one member immediately affects others, and stress in an individual member reverberates strongly across the boundaries and is swiftly echoed in other subsystems" (Minuchin, 1974, p. 55). The concepts of time, force, and reverberation, all part of general systems theory, are crucial to understanding the enmeshed family and its opposite, the disengaged family. In the disengaged family, interpersonal distance is too great; the boundaries between subsystems are rigid; and the reverberating potential is low. While a single minor event, such as a child's sneeze, is sufficient in the enmeshed family to produce instant and immense medical attention from both parents, the disengaged family can tolerate large individual pathologies with scarcely a notice. In one disengaged family, for example, a teenage son had been in jail for three days following a drug arrest. The parents had been unaware and unconcerned about his absence from the home, thinking he was simply coming home late at night and leaving early in the morning before other family members were up. Examples of enmeshed family members abound, especially in reports of families with highly disturbed children. In one enmeshed family with a diagnosed schizophrenic son, the mother and father daily weighed both the food the child ate and the stool he produced, showing great concern if there was a discrepancy between the two weights. Following Minuchin's diagrammatic notations, these boundary pathologies are depicted in Figure 2-1.

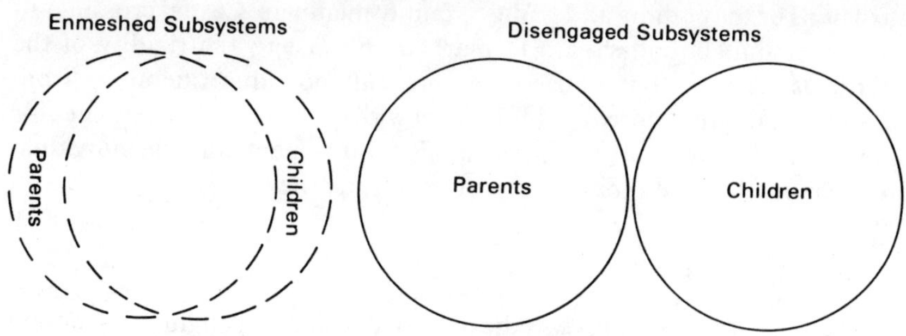

FIGURE 2-1. A diagrammatic representation of subsystem boundary pathologies.

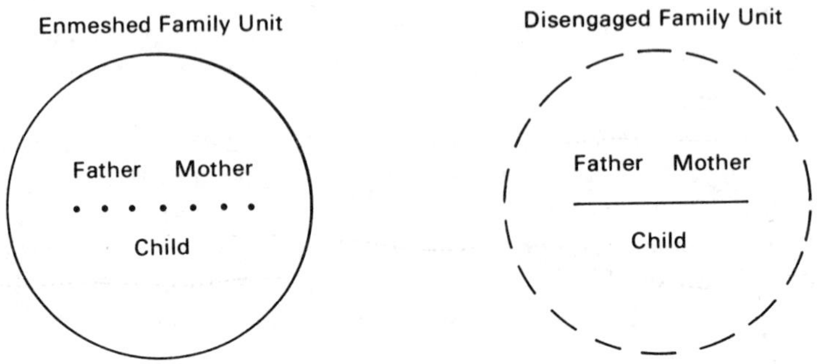

FIGURE 2-2. Troubled alliance behavior in the two extremes of boundary pathology.

Troubled boundaries are the subsystem expression of troubled alliances among family members. In the enmeshed family, parents and children are likely to be overinvolved, while in the disengaged family, they have too little to do with each other. These two family types can be further characterized with regard to their family-unit boundary, a perspective that makes even more clear the possibility for troubled alliance behavior.

The family-unit boundary of the enmeshed family is often rigid and closed, tending to shut out the external world and to imprison its members, holding them captive to the entanglements of the subsystems that, conversely, are too diffusely bounded to promote individual autonomy (see Fig. 2-2). When there is an absence of appropriate and clear boundaries between family members and when the potentially corrective contact of the outside world is denied, then the alliances between family members are too tight. This yields an exaggerated sense of belonging to the family group and too little autonomous sense of simply being oneself. The disengaged family, on the other hand, has a family-unit boundary that is far too diffuse to offer a comfortable regulation of either society's intrusions or the coming and going of family members. Casual crossings of this larger unit boundary are in marked contrast to the rigidity of the internal subsystem boundaries that prevent individual members from having meaningful or predictable contact with each other. Too few cues for identity and behavior are available in this arrangement, and the individual members may seek definition in groups outside the family.

Pathology of Alliances

The structural view reveals the pattern of splits and alignments among family members and thereby provides an emphasis on affiliations. Family structure consists of both the alliances and the antagonisms among members as well as the boundaries creating durable subsystems. Just as there can be pathologies of the boundary, so too can there be alliance pathologies. There are two principal types of alliance pathology: conflict detouring or scapegoating and inappropriate cross-generational coalitions.

In alliances that achieve conflict detouring, one finds the clinically familiar pattern of two parents who express a total absence of conflict between themselves but are instead solidly united against an individual child or subunit of children. Conflict detouring reduces pressure on the spouse subsystem, but clearly places stress upon the children. Clinicians often have difficulty dealing with this arrangement. They too readily sympathize with the scapegoated child, often making an alliance with the child that then prevents the family from mounting its own rescue actions, an event that would reveal valuable data about their structural arrangements.

Patterns of detouring and scapegoating are generally easier to recognize than those of cross-generational coalitions. Whether covert or overt, these coalitions typically begin with one parent and a child in a tightly bounded antagonism toward the other parent—for example, a mother that successfully forces her son into a union of continual, though perhaps covert, reproach to the father. (See Fig. 2-3.)

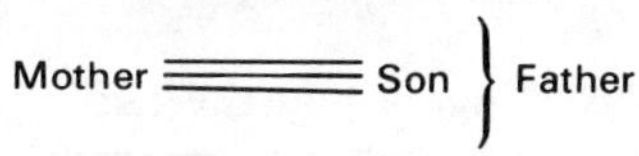

FIGURE 2-3. An example of cross-generational coalition.

These coalitions may come to include others or even all of the remaining family members. Note that a critical term here is *cross-generational.* When the coalition (an arrangement that is challenging and combative in its inevitable opposition to some third party) involves a cross-generational alliance, then the result is generally pathological. Naturally, one refers here to coalitions that have endured over a considerable time and around a variety of family themes; temporary coalitions formed to pursue limited goals are exempted from any pathological connotation.

Pathology of Triangles

Both detouring and cross-generational coalitions are specific forms of triangulation. Each arrangement tends to pit two family members against a third, though other family members may join either side. Along with Caplow (1968), the structuralists have suggested that triangles are inherently unstable, tending periodically to resolve themselves into arrangements of two against one. When the two consists of both parents,

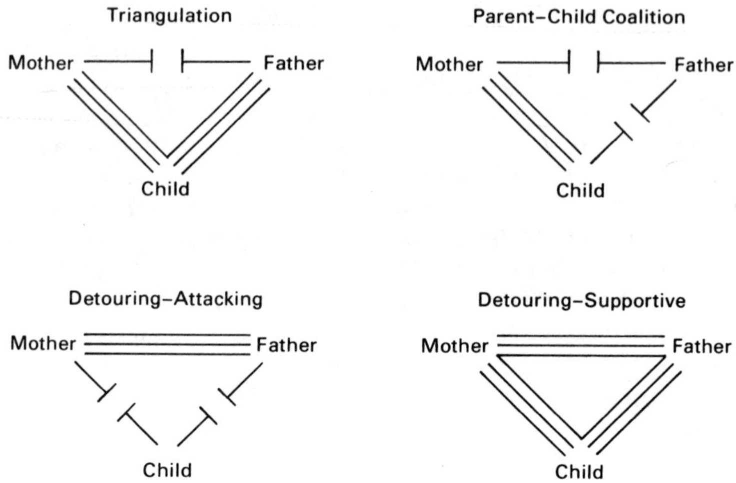

FIGURE 2-4. Four pathological triangles showing how family conflict is detoured, concealed, or expressed via cross-generational coalitions. [Adapted from Minuchin, S., Roseman, B. L., & Baker, L. *Psychosomatic families: Anorexia nervosa in context.* Cambridge, Massachusetts: Harvard University Press, 1978.]

we find instances of detouring. When the two consists of a parent plus child, we find instances of cross-generational alliances. One may, of course, argue that dyads are also inherently unstable and become stable only when in a state of triangulation; that is, only when their subunit boundary is clearly defined by the presence of an excluded third person. Either way, this alliance structure, if it endures long enough, brings heavy penalties to both sides, and symptomatic behavior will occur.

These instances of misalliance, as well as matters of hierarchical imbalance, can also be presented in terms of disturbed triangles. In their work with psychosomatic families, Minuchin, Roseman, and Baker (1978) presented a typology of *rigid triads.* Beginning with the hypothesis that children could be used to conceal or deflect parental conflict, they described four triadic arrangements that increased the likelihood of symptomatic behavior in the child. These are presented in Figure 2-4. Lynn Hoffman has recently offered a succinct summary of these arrangements:

> "Triangulation" describes a situation where two parents, in overt or covert conflict, are each attempting to enlist the child's sympathy or support against the other . . . [this is a] triangle with two positive sides, connoting intense conflict of loyalty. "Parent–Child" is a more open expression of parental conflict, even though the family may come for treatment with a child problem. One parent will side with the child against the other parent, and at

> times it is difficult to determine whether the child or the outsider spouse is in more difficulty. The intense closeness of the child to the preferred parent can result in symptomatology, however, especially when the natural process of growing up begins to put stress on the parent–child stasis. There are two types of "Detouring" triads. In a "Detouring-Attacking" triad, the parents are most often perceived by the clinician as scapegoating the child. The behavior the child shows is disruptive or "bad," and the parents band together to control him, even though one parent is often apt to disagree with the other parent over how to handle him and both may handle him inconsistently. Most behavior disorders in children fall into this category. In a "Detouring-Supportive" triad the parents are able to mask their differences by focusing on a child who is defined as "sick," and for whom the parents show an enormous, overprotective concern. This brings them close together and is a frequent feature of families in which tension is expressed through psychosomatic disorders. All these triads . . . can be found in families with psychosomatic children, but they are prevalent in families where children have other problems as well (1981, pp.150–151).

Pathology of Hierarchies

The inversion of power hierarchies is often labeled as the single most destructive force in a family's structure. Haley has, in fact, implicated it as the chief source of trouble in his recent book on treating highly disturbed youth (1980). In one sense, hierarchical difficulties are a special form of alliance pathologies, as when a mother and child form the parental subunit, excluding the father. Such inversions, however, often occur not in a dyadic alliance, but in situations where only a single person is involved. When, for example, a father loses his job and the mother is forced to work, many hierarchical imbalances occur: the father may be at home taking a more nurturant role with the children while the mother is out at work, struggling with all the pressures of full employment. Most would agree that this state of affairs creates a difference, but whether it creates pathology depends on the strength with which the traditional, middle-class culture has left its mark on the family. If the family completely subscribes to a stereotyped pattern of normality, and/or if the surrounding culture gives little support for such role reversals, then father-as-housewife and mother-as-breadwinner may indeed become an hierarchy inversion that leads to family trouble.

Somewhat less value-laden are judgments about families run by the children. When executive power has been surrendered to a child, as may often be observed in families with children characterized by severe medical or psychological distress, then dysfunctional behavior appears in nearly all subunits of the family system. Such an arrangement cannot long endure within the family and, most certainly, cannot allow the family to cope with demands from outside the family; children do not pay bills, negotiate educational routines, or make medical decisions. Parents do, at least in our culture. Consequently, there is a therapeutic emphasis on correcting a disabling power hierarchy before moving on to other areas of family life.

A SYSTEMS VIEW OF FAMILY THERAPY

Minuchin and Fishman (1981) presented two views of the therapeutic effort: one humanistic (something previously felt lacking in structural family therapies) and one systemic. In a philosophically positive way, they argued that the good therapist helps the family discover new realities about its collective identity. There is a poetical expansion of life possibilities as the constraints of context are transformed into opportunities for new and creative alteration of family image. The strengths and possibilities for any family are not unlimited, but they are most assuredly larger than most people usually experience.

Aside from this poetical view of change, when Minuchin and Fishman returned to a systems orientation, they recognized that a troubled family is stuck in a dysfunctional homeostatic phase. Therefore, the therapist must ". . . move the family to a stage of creative turmoil where what was given must be replaced by a search for new ways. Flexibility must be induced by increasing the system's fluctuations, ultimately moving it toward a higher level of complexity" (1981, p.27). To transform the system, it must first be unbalanced. Where there is no crisis, there is no need for alternatives; where alternatives are missing, there is no complexity; and where complexity is absent, there is no growth, only unhappy stagnation. The structural therapist understands that the experience of any subsystem is, as Minuchin and Fishman have noted, ". . . constrained by the contextual structure. Therefore, breaking or expanding contexts can allow new possibilities to emerge. The therapist, an expander of contexts, creates a context in which exploration of the unfamiliar is possible" (p.15). The concepts of crisis, flux, new homeostatic stabilities, and the alternation of individual with family change combine to create a plan for structural change.

A PLAN FOR STRUCTURAL CHANGE

The goal of structural interventions should be the repositioning of individual family members within their primary and secondary subsystems, with an attendant opportunity to form new and healthier alliances and structures. The repositioning of individuals and the subsequent emergence of new structures should benefit the index patient as well as the entire family. Both the presenting problem and the "redefined problem" should be substantially improved. Structural interventions should also enable the family to move into states of more complex systems functioning rather than remain in the less complex, often rigid structural patterns characteristic of disturbed families. When more complex and differentiated systems behavior has been achieved, the structural interventions will have facilitated the family's adaptation to its life-cycle task. Minuchin and Fishman, in agreement with this notion of change, have made these comments:

> The structural approach sees the family as an organism: a complex system that is underfunctioning. The therapist undermines the existing homeostasis, creating crises that jar the system toward the development of a better functioning organization . . . the old order must be undermined to allow for the formation of the new (p. 67).

Their tactics of change require the therapist to challenge the presenting symptom, the family structure, and the family reality, the superordinate world view that organizes many of the family's perceptions and values. Ultimately, for Minuchin and Fishman, the goal of structural change is always ". . . the conversion of the family to a different world-view—one that does not need the symptom—and to a more flexible, pluralistic view of reality—one that allows for diversity within a more complex universe" (p.215).

Implicit in these theoretical and ideal definitions of change are certain processes whereby structural change may occur. The process of structural change involves three overlapping objectives: (1) to challenge the prevailing homeostatic norms in order to (2) introduce crisis and flux in the system, an instability that will position people to behave and feel differently about themselves and each other and (3) thereby to develop new behavioral routines or sequences that make up the new system structures. The evolution of these new structural arrangements occurs when new behavioral sequences are repeated over time and with emotional force.

Each new structural arrangement may be a preparation for yet another stage in the change process or may be a temporary end in itself. Many structural arrangements are simply the best possible ones at that time and, as such, are necessary steps towards more functional levels of family organization. Other structural rearrangements may be more durable, enjoying healthy homeostatic flux as they regulate longer periods of the family's life cycle.

The cycle of structural change may take families through several such transitional stages until they reach a level of family organization that relieves them of the presenting problems. Figure 2-5 illustrates this general plan for structural change.

The following are the important features presented in Figure 2-5. First, not only is there obvious movement through time, but graphically this movement is "upward," connoting a shift from more static and rigid organizational structures to ones of greater energy and diversity. Second, this movement alternates between periods of a system's flux (morphogenetic phase) with periods of relative equilibrium (morphostatic phase).

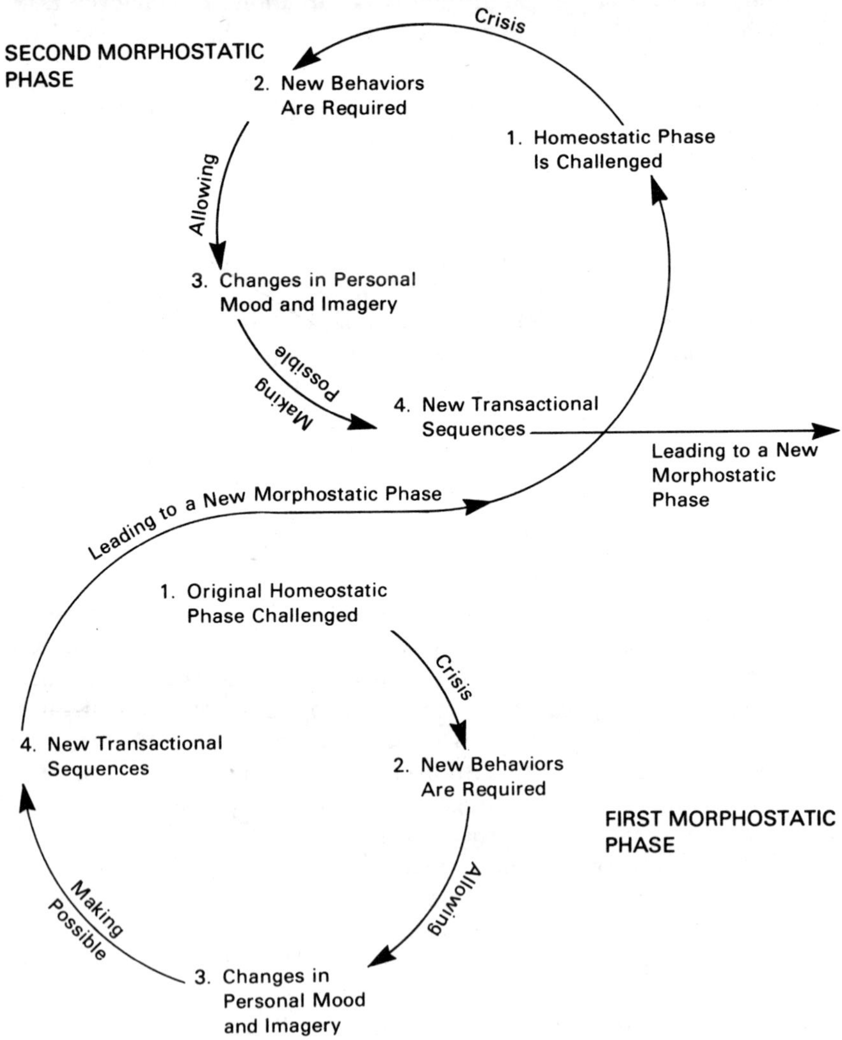

FIGURE 2-5. A plan for structural change in a normal adaptive system.

The duration of each phase depends, on the one hand, on the family's capacity to bear conflict and crisis and, on the other hand, the helpfulness or harm of remaining in a state of near equilibrium. Matters of duration are always an issue of judgment and inevitability; skilled therapists need to recognize when a family has wisely settled into a period of calm and to make such judgments. They also must accept the powerful and often inevitable capacity of a family to foreshorten periods of crisis, preferring instead the covert pathologies of prolonged periods of stasis. The determination of when enough is enough, whether in reference to change or to calm, naturally varies with the goals of each case.

Third, this simplified plan for change can be easily identified in terms of its components:

1. The therapist intervenes with the prevailing homeostatic arrangement in a way that creates crisis or flux.
2. This crisis requires people to behave in new ways, something the therapist encourages.
3. New behavior allows the family members to have new feelings and images about themselves. This is a part of the cybernetic loop connecting each individual to the larger group.
4. New behaviors and new images make possible the emergence of new transactional sequences among family members. Because these new sequences occur within the forming constraints of a living system, there is a great likelihood they will be repeated and will become part of the family's routine.
5. The consequences of such repetition are the formation of a new set of structures and a new plateau of equilibrium.

As noted, whether there is movement through another cycle of change or whether the family rests where it is depends on the family's life-cycle needs and on the status of the presenting problems. Typically, families go through a very small number of such cycles during the course of therapy.

This brief sketch of a plan for change is intended only as a rough guide to clinical intervention, not as a theoretical description of how change may actually occur. The dynamics of change are extraordinarily complex, and there is no single viewpoint that is overwhelmingly persuasive. Structural family therapy proceeds *as if* change flowed through a spiral of cycles like those diagrammed above; but the procedure is argued primarily as a guide to therapists who understandably require some larger sense of direction. In fact, recent work by Hoffman (1980, 1981) and others has suggested that change occurs not continuously, but rather through a kind of "evolutionary leap," wherein the system is quite suddenly transformed. Whatever the ultimate dynamics of change may be, structural therapists design their interventions to create cycles of crisis and stability, finding that model a good enough guide for everyday clinical practice.

SYMBOLS OF STRUCTURAL DIAGNOSIS

In the examples so far given, diagrams of lines and spatial arrangements convey information about the family's structure. This technique of depicting family structure through diagrams is useful in concretizing early diagnostic assumptions and in planning the treatment procedure. These diagrams, usually referred to as a *systems map* or a *structural map,* have been described by Minuchin:

> A family map is an organizational scheme. It does not represent the richness of family transactions any more than a map represents the richness of a territory. It is static, whereas the family is constantly in motion. But the family map is a powerful simplification device, which allows the therapist to organize the diverse material that he is getting. The map allows him to formulate hypotheses about areas within the family that function well and about other areas that may be dysfunctional. It also helps him determine therapeutic goals (1974, p.90).

Minuchin (1974) has offered a series of symbols useful in the mapping process. They may be rearranged and extended in the following ways.

Boundaries

As noted earlier, the boundaries of any system are the rules defining who participates in it and the degree of access outsiders have to the system. These rule governed behaviors create three types of boundaries:

1. A *clear* or *open* boundary, represented by dashes: --------
2. A *closed* or *rigid* boundary, represented by a solid line: ________
3. A *diffuse* boundary, represented by dots: • • • •

These boundary lines may be drawn around the entire family unit. For example, a family-unit boundary that is closed would appear this way:

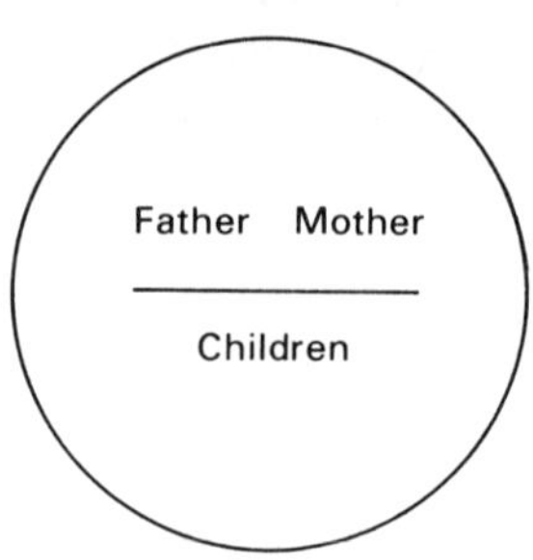

These boundary lines may also be placed between the smaller subsystems within the total family unit. This placement will emphasize an interface quality between the two units. For example, an open boundary between the parental and sibling subsystems would be designated as such:

Father Mother

\- - - - - - -

Children

Alliances and Affiliations

Map symbols can also be used to depict the quality of *usual* transactions between two family members:

1. A clear and friendly alliance of presumed normal nature is depicted by a double line. For example, a normal bond between spouses would be indicated this way:

   Husband ═══ Wife

2. An enmeshed or overinvolved affiliation is depicted by three lines. An overinvolved, cross-generation bond would, for example, appear as such:

   Mother ≡≡≡ Son

3. A weak or unknown affiliation is depicted by dots, as shown below:

   Father . . . . Daughter

4. A conflicted affiliation, e.g., a sibling conflict, is designated by this symbol:

   Sister ——| |—— Brother

5. A coalition of several family members against another member, or against several other members is depicted by brackets. The example below shows the mother and two daughters in coalition against father and son:

   Mother
Daughter } { Father
Daughter Son

Detouring Conflict

A frequent observation is that two family members preserve their relationship by detouring incipient conflict through some third person.

For example, a father and mother, both stressed at work, may avoid attacking each other at home by uniting in an attack on their child, thereby detouring conflict between themselves. This detouring is shown by the symbol:

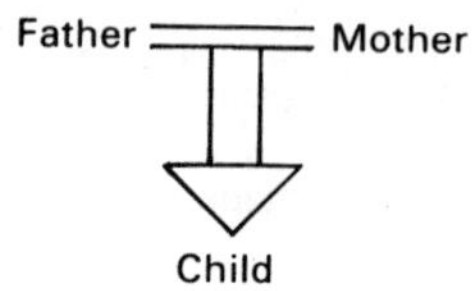

Mapping Strategies

Mapping the family system offers two diagnostic advantages. It helps describe how the entire family is organized, and it can also describe the particular subunit that is most involved in a problem. (See Figs. 2–6 and 2–7.)

Structural maps are useful in helping to organize family process data into some elementary guesses about the structural features of the family. The maps should be quickly revised or discarded as new data appears. Therapists should practice making such maps, but they should also be ready to revise them as new information emerges.

The remainder of this book is about how to implement a structural plan for change. It is a guide to how one arranges a setting so that a family may break its old contextual constraints, enter some temporary state of crisis, and then achieve a new, more complex reality about life's possibilities.

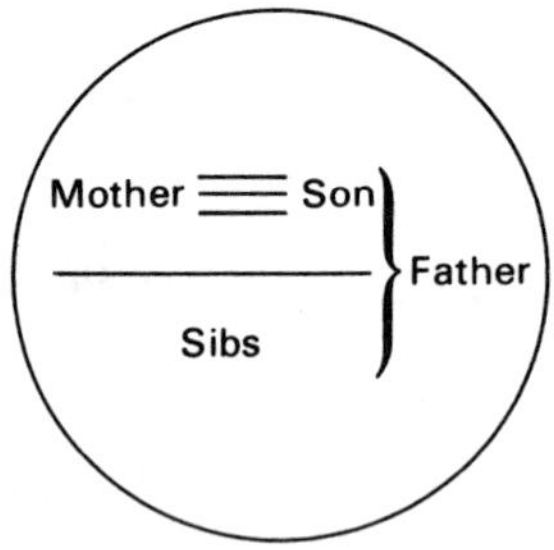

FIGURE 2-6. This diagram shows a closed-family-unit boundary with an overinvolved mother and son comprising the parental subsystem. Between them and the other children is a rigid boundary, yet apparently under enough control so that all are in a coalition against the father.

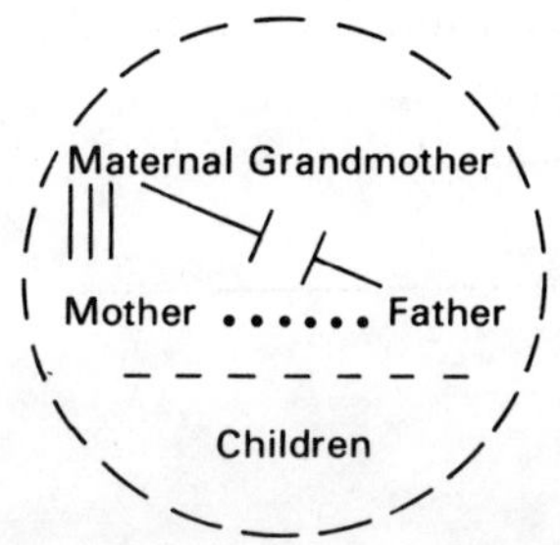

FIGURE 2-7. This map shows an open-family-unit boundary, enclosing a parental subsystem characterized by the mother's overinvolvement with her own mother, who in turn is in conflict with her daughter's husband, perhaps related to the diffuse tie between the spouses. The map also shows a normal open boundary between parents and children.

Chapter 3

Joining and Diagnosis

To join a family group means to contact it and then to experience the vicissitudes of contact, the myriad ways in which this contact is embraced, resisted, and reciprocated by the family as a unit and by the individual members. How the family system accommodates to this event—the approach of the therapist—offers one key diagnostic information about prominent features of family functioning. As Minuchin has said, "Diagnosis in family therapy is achieved through the interactional process of joining" (1974, p.130).

The therapist joins primarily through contact with individual family members, not with some abstraction called the "system," although some properties of the superordinate entity, such as mood, tempo, language, will soon emerge, and these will influence the therapist's joining style. But in the beginning, one meets individuals, experiencing with each of them intimations of affinity or hostility, which contribute to an emotional field that will expel or admit the therapist to various parts of the family system. The process of contact and response to contact is inevitable since to join a family is of necessity to interfere with its life. Joining is an effort to cross the family-unit boundary, gaining a foothold wherever possible, seeking alliances with any subgroup willing to make one. This interference in the family's life, however benevolent in intention, will naturally be examined, resisted, incorporated, and when possible, reframed in terms of the family's values about nonfamily individuals. These struggles around contact with the therapist occur not randomly, but in patterns. The act of joining is thus an act of discovering the system's secrets, of experiencing and perceiving its patterned way of admitting newness (the therapist) to its life. In this way, *the act of joining is an act of diagnosis.*

Joining is partly a matter of fitting in, of finding out how the family does its business, and then, at times, of choosing to conform to those rules. But joining as a diagnostic strategy also requires one to attempt an alteration of those rules and then to observe how the family reacts. The therapist may find intelligent and sympathetic ways of joining that maintain a family's status quo; this yields some diagnostic information, but of a lesser value than those therapist behaviors designed to challenge and change some part of the system. Put this way, joining a family is not simply some innocent social gesture or some variation on building rapport between client and therapist. On the contrary, joining as a concept embodies a distinct notion about the diagnostic procedure—namely, that an accurate and *therapeutically useful* systems diagnosis emerges primarily through efforts to alter the system one is joining. This view of diagnosis stands in considerable contrast to more traditional diagnostic procedures, which assume that a therapist may observe the client as a psychosocial entity immune to the consequences of this observation. The client, it is presumed, will reside in this state of innocent immunity until, following a compilation of diagnostic impressions and tests, some therapeutic procedure is later applied. What distinguishes the systems-oriented perspective is a diagnosis achieved through observation of the family's response to treatment interventions; then, in circular fashion, there is revision of the initial formulations and subsequent treatment steps, all such alterations occurring in a relatively continuous, spiraling succession of therapist and family interactions. It is not the family as some static entity that is diagnosed; instead, it is the family's interactive process with the therapist, an agent of change, that becomes the focus of the diagnostic experience.

DIAGNOSIS AND THERAPIST ACTIVITY

This definition of diagnosis signals the absence of traditional therapist neutrality and the presence of a good deal of therapist activity. Such a diagnostic approach avoids a Newtonian subject–object dichotomy and replaces it with notions of circular causality, which, when combined with general systems theory, make it necessary for the therapist to become involved in activating the family's feedback loops and in eliciting the covert structures that govern family life. Opponents of such therapist activity have widely misunderstood its intent, thinking of it as primarily an authoritarian stance used by unsophisticated, beginning therapists. On the other hand, its proponents often substitute a good deal of seat-of-the-pants nonsense for careful diagnostic assessments, substituting busy-ness for accurate observations about the family's collective behavior.

Activity in one's joining techniques involves two points: first, that no stranger crosses into the life of a family without encountering its rules for admission; and, second, that such a stranger should, nonetheless, not hesitate to knock at the family's door. The hesitation to knock too often characterizes many traditional diagnostic procedures, though breaking down the door will hardly give the systems-oriented therapist any valuable information. How the therapist knocks, who in the family answers the door, and in what manner, are the chief issues when joining is a key to diagnosis.

Joining: Ways to Knock

There are both formal and informal ways to describe a therapist's joining activity. The informal way refers to the personal style and stance assumed by a therapist upon endeavoring to join and change the family. As therapists are meddlers by necessity, not uninvolved and neutral scientists, matters of personal style are crucial and point to the means by which therapists use themselves to create the affiliation necessary for the family to benefit from therapeutic meddling in its life. Occasionally, this acknowledgement of personal involvement in those transactions that influence a family is taken as an encouragement to speak of the "use of self" as though "self" were some grand new tool discovered by family therapists. Indeed, some therapists, perhaps in a mistaken effort to counter the fabled (though generally illusory) neutrality of the psychoanalytic therapist, seem to burden their clients with personal revelations about themselves. This is the "use of self" that constitutes a misuse of the other person.

To be one's self with a family does not mean that one has to be personally revealing or openly striving to establish some sense of sameness with the client. Some similarities will naturally exist, but the inevitable differences between each person—the distinctive colorations that make each of us unique from the other—are of greater use to the therapist who is joining a new system. To know what is personally distinct about oneself (however one comes to learn this) will include knowing how one characteristically enters new systems. When therapists know and appreciate the diverse and wonderful complexities of who they are as individuals, then they have many options for how to enter any particular family. For example, therapists who know something about themselves and their own family background will be informed in their moves into families that are quite like their own as compared to those families that are quite different. Very simply, to "use one's self" in therapy only means to be oneself and to be personally clear about one's way of being-in-systems. To know one's best moves into new systems and then to make them without great fanfare is a good enough use of self in the therapeutic process.

Quite aside from the marvelous differences among family therapists, an infinitude of variance that cannot be catalogued, there are some idealized constellations of behavior that might be called a therapist's stance. Several such stances are useful both in joining and throughout the therapy. While these have only the status of nominal descriptions and none of the elegance of a theoretical prescription, they are helpful guides when thinking about the roles available when one finds oneself at work.

Stances

ENTRY: PINBALL MACHINES AND THE SCIENTIFIC PLAYER. The family, like the pinball machine, is an elaborate design for wins and losses, combined under some unifying rubric intended to attract continual play. Whether the system calls itself "Roller Queen" or "This Family Wins at Everything," what, or who, enters it may have the qualities of an unexpected outsider: a steel ball in the case of the pinball machine and a therapist in the case of the troubled family. From the viewpoint of a systems tinker, one meddling in the mechanics of relatedness, a therapist can be a novel event, an entity not included in the original design but who nonetheless drops into play. Like the steel ball, therapists may enter this prearranged system with varying degrees of force, depending on their individual styles of play and the boundaries of the family unit. And like the systems scientists they are, therapists, having made the play and the entrance, then watch to see how the system, when left to its own devices, will process them. In pinball, this would take the unheard-of form of simply shooting in the ball and then watching it race around, without any interference from the shooter, to carom off interfaces, score, rebound, and finally vanish, leaving the machine humming but essentially the same.

Having made enough of these observations, the player-therapist moves on to the real game, that of shooting into the system interventions designed to violate the natural order of things. Now the effort is to provoke a higher score—using side flippers and body blows—but without precipitating a tilt. In a cool way, therapists may observe the family as a natural system that metabolizes their inputs and may stand scientific watch as the family either struggles to digest these inputs or is forced to redesign some aspect of its system in order to accommodate to the new player. This must all be done without a trace of tilt, or the game is over.

The pinball metaphor is helpful as long as it is not mistaken for a permanent position. If it is, one is aspiring to the observational neutrality of science, which in itself is a myth but which is nevertheless seductively persuasive to therapists who fear an emotional commitment of themselves to the fray. That is the danger of this particular stance. Its advantages, however, are many, not the least of which is a chance finally to become an anthropologist visiting a small society and silently observing its rules for making something of this person who has dropped into its midst and who insists, with many questions and comments, on zinging from one boundary to another, ringing bells, lighting up markers, and forever driving up the ante of the game.

INDUCTION: THE CONVERT. There is nothing like being a convert to discover the evils of conversion and the constraints of belief. A good therapist may join a family by occasionally converting to its folkways. In matters of tone, idiom, and gesture, the therapist will follow the rules of this congregation in order to experience truly the rigors of family faith. This stance is especially helpful in the opening sessions, when the family wants to take the therapist in, but only if the therapist agrees to be like its family members. It is a troublesome stance if there is no sinful intention in the therapist's heart, since only a private determination to break the rules of the group will prevent the therapist's baptism from becoming an induction. Induction is one's unwitting conformance to the family's pathological process and structures. Therapists accept the fact that at times induction is simply the inevitable price of joining, but they also cultivate the confidence that total subscription to the family's rituals is unlikely. Otherwise, they would not be therapists at all, but only grownups looking for conversion. Complete induction renders the therapist quite useless as an agent of change and is the danger of volunteering for baptism. Some assume that being inducted is a painful process and that the pain itself will help the therapist recognize when induction has taken place. Unhappily, as the following example shows (Umbarger & Hare, 1973), when joining becomes induction, the therapist is usually the last to know.

The Decker family. The Deckers sought help because of the persistently peculiar behavior of Eddie, their 12-year-old son, who had been diagnosed as schizophrenic.* He had many bizarre mannerisms, speech that was often incoherent, an odd posture and gait, many fears, and numerous somatic complaints. On the other hand, he was of normal intelligence and had some friends. He attended a public school where his work was flawed but not hopeless. Nonetheless, his sticky enmeshment with his parents (he was their only child) put narrow and stringent limits on his development, and he seemed, as adolescence approached, increasingly immature and inappropriate in his behavior. During the preceding four

---

*This case history of the Decker family is modified from Umbarger, C., & Hare, R. A structural approach to patient and therapist disengagement from a schizophrenic family. *American Journal of Psychotherapy,* 1973, *27,* 274–284. With permission.

years, the family had defeated a variety of therapeutic efforts. The following excerpt, a reconstruction of taped interviews, shows how difficult it was to escape conversion to their family religion.

Harry and Imogene Decker seemed to costume themselves for the role of patients. Their outfits, down to the smallest detail, were comic parodies of a dress style fashionable only for the back wards of state mental hospitals. Theirs was a kind of chronic chic. Imogene, a small woman, wore pink sweatsocks, blowzy skirts of indeterminate age and style, and mismatched blouses. Harry, a heavy man, was less floridly dressed, yet there was an unmistakable air of cultivated defiance about his clothes. His grey workpants, always several sizes too large, were bunched together at his waist by a beaded Indian belt. Like Imogene, he carried at least one paper shopping bag and sometimes two, filled with items that were indispensable only for a person going on the bum in an unfriendly climate: extra socks, woolen scarfs, a foreign language dictionary, and a box of Girl Scout cookies.

In the midst of the shuffle of parental shopping bags was Eddie. He was tall, ungainly, yet delicately made, a marionette whose strings were of the wrong length. He spoke in a high, rapid voice, sometimes slurring his words so badly that even the most practiced and patient parent would have difficulty understanding him.

Therapy sessions inevitably began with this small family of three dividing themselves into two whirlwind armies who would descend on the therapist from opposite ends of the corridor. With gales of strained laughter, they would finally enter the therapy room.

"I might choke to death," said Imogene, "since this room seems filled with chalk dust. Too much erasing, not enough correctness." She settled into one chair, then tried another, looking suspiciously under each chair for some evidence of dust and dirt. Harry was solicitous, though uneasy with his wife's behavior. He offered to change seats with her, made a few ineffectual efforts to clean the blackboard, and then returned to his seat.

"There's dust at school, too," volunteered Eddie.

"Tell the doctor what happened there, if he wants to know," Mr. Decker said.

The therapist, feeling that a direction and topic were emerging, readily agreed. "By all means. What happened?" He was unaware that he had fallen in with Harry and Eddie, who were effectively diverting attention from Imogene's odd behavior by introducing Eddie's school problems.

Eddie stared intently at his mother, never losing eye contact with her as he told his story. "I fell on the playground and scraped my side. Then when I got to the nurse's office, I thought I might faint from the algebra left to do, so naturally I made the nurse call my mother and then I went home.

And that's all of that. Aside from the three tongues." So saying, he seemed to consider the matter closed, although Mrs. Decker clearly had more on her mind.

"Thank God, I was at home, the streets being what they are. Boy Scouts or no Boy Scouts," she concluded as a kind of mysterious afterthought.

"I think we should get down to an efficient discussion of why we are coming here, not why there are no Boy Scouts on the streets." Mr. Decker was again responding to his wife's meanderings by trying to organize the family.

"I thought we settled that last year," replied Mrs. Decker, "when we were worried about how Eddie was picked on in school. And his dizzy spells, some of which must be due to all the dust that's around."

"Is that what you've been worried about all this time?" asked Harry. "I thought you wondered about the fatigue of your mental processes and why your feet are swelling."

"Mother's feet don't swell," said Eddie, heading off any focus on his mother.

"I'm sorry," Harry grinned weakly.

"Why can't you be wrong like other men without having to be sorry all the time?" Mrs. Decker said. "Then our social life would improve."

The therapist, losing track of the bewildering school problems, moved quickly in support of Mrs. Decker's new topic. "Are you asking your husband to change something about your social life?" Although well intended, the question supported an implicit criticism of Mr. Decker and ignored his efforts of only a moment ago to "organize" the discussion, a typical fate for Mr. Decker's efforts to be efficient. As the therapist slipped from side to side, first in alliance with efforts to ignore Mrs. Decker's concern with a dusty, poisonous environment and then with *her* efforts to ignore Mr. Decker's attempt at organizing the family, he got a premonition of the trip to come.

Mrs. Decker grew wistful for a second. "We used to go to parties all the time, but the person who invited us died."

"I asked you to go to a meeting of Radicals-Over-Thirty with me and you refused. You complained that political people don't know how to polka. I mean I tried." Harry seemed genuinely hurt by his wife's attack.

The therapist, trying to hold onto a topic, said, "Each of you seems to really want the same thing, to do something together socially." He skipped over Harry's hurt feeling, inadvertently supporting Mrs. Decker's injunction that her husband should stop feeling "sorry" every time he was criticized. The family "rule" that mother should never be found wanting was being scrupulously, though inadvertently, observed by the therapist.

Just to make sure, Imogene flared up, scooting to the edge of her chair. "Are you implying that we are a failure of social ethics?"

"Etiquette," said Harry.

"Ethical societies don't interest us and never will," Imogene continued. "Moreover, there is nothing funny about trying to be ethical, and I resent your implication that my husband and I aren't ethical."

"I only suggested that the two of you might do something social together . . . that is, not separate. Ah, thinking for the future . . . that is, since the past is over." The therapist was uncomfortable, but still trying to give cogent meanings to the conversation and smooth over ruffled feelings, a response typical of outsiders who tried to get inside this family.

"Mommy and Daddy can't go out," whined Eddie, "I need them at home to help me with my merit badges." He too was sitting on the edge of his chair, eyes fastened on his mother, with a glazed look, as if transported by a thought of a merit badge in social ethics.

Suddenly, on some secret signal, all three members of the family arose and, crossing impolitely in front of the therapist, switched seats, each person moving over one chair.

"Whenever I stand up in here, the room gets small," said Eddie in his *Alice in Wonderland* voice.

"Then sit down!" replied the harassed therapist. He relaxed, happily unaware that he sounded just like one of the family.

"What is the rationale for peephole therapy?" asked Imogene, apparently referring to the observation mirror along one side of the room.

"Whatever it is," replied Harry in his efficient voice, while pulling a thermos from his shopping bag, "I think it's time for a tea break."

"It's always the same here," sighed Eddie, taking a small wax cup of tepid tea. "Nothing ever changes, week after week."

"Better safe than sorry," commented Mrs. Decker dramatically.

"Precisely how many weeks has it been?" said Mr. Decker, still dreaming of organization.

"Thirteen," said the therapist, holding out his cup.

TAKING CHARGE: DIRECTORS AND SCRIPTS. Unlike the *auteur* film director who simultaneously directs and writes the script, family therapists should assume a stance of directing, but leave the *latent* script to the family. Latent is emphasized because the script being played daily seems utterly awful and deserves nothing but the worst of critical reviews. Hence, some therapists may assume that they need to write an entirely new play for the family. This is not only impolite and often impossible, but ignores the likelihood that if one bothers to look, the family has a script in mind, a good one, but needs obvious help in the production. The family is not, as some suggest, analogous to "six characters in search of an author." However amateurishly, most family groups have already rehearsed a new and better script than the one they play each day. This is true of even the most disturbed families who, given the right inquiry, show surprising amounts of sophistication about the changes needed in their show. Consequently, the danger of this stance is that the therapist presumes to write the story when all that is required is rather firm direction of a family script too long postponed.

The advantage of this stance is that it allows the therapist to assume, in a straightforward manner, the leadership rightfully invested in a therapist. The family comes for help because it has not solved its own problems and has consequently agreed to hire the therapist to provide new directions. This stance is not just one stance interchangeable with many others, depending upon the momentary needs of the therapy, but rather a general and enduring attitude toward one's therapeutic presence. Leadership is required, and the therapist who fails to take it openly, and thereby comfortably, is destined to take it covertly and by default. The therapist, as Minuchin (Minuchin & Fishman, 1981) has noted, is an "expander of contexts," a person who actively suggests to the family alternative ways of regarding reality and of behaving within its own system, in accordance with a script that the family has already begun. In taking this leadership, the therapist forms a new unit, that of family *plus* therapist, within which changes can occur.

In 1981, Minuchin and Fishman added other classifications of joining moves, using "different positions of proximity." They listed three positions arrayed on an implicit continuum of emotional involvement and supportiveness. In the *close position*, therapists are supportive and nurturant; they reflect back to the family an understanding of its pain and allow themselves to be inducted into the family's view of reality. They form affiliations and consistently confirm the family's emotions and ideational stands, always striving to find the positive connotation to the family's actions. By reserving the power to confirm others, the therapist develops leverage with the family.

A step away is the *median position* in which the therapist joins as an active but neutral listener. Minuchin and Fishman called this modality "tracking," a consistent attentiveness to helping people develop the details of their story. From this position, the therapist not only helps the family elaborate the many consequences of its life routines, but also begins interventions, usually into the process aspects of the family's behavior rather than the content of the family's stories. "Tracking means not only to follow but also gently to direct explorations of new behavior. It means to shift levels of tracking from content to process . . ." (p.38).

The *disengaged position* finds the therapist still in a neutral emotional stance, but very directive in the interventions. Like the "pinball player," the therapist has not only observed the "patterns of the family dance" (Minuchin & Fishman, p.40), but now actively applies pressure to alter the routines. The therapist creates new contexts for behavior by directing people in novel scenarios of interaction, bringing together, for example, family members who usually avoid each other. Unlike the close position in which the therapist is very much the "sympathetic relative," in this position the therapist joins by being an expert director of change.

Joining is an affiliative act that leads to both diagnosis and change and then renewed diagnosis. Although emphasized at the beginning of contact with a family, it occurs in every stage of treatment.

TYPES OF THERAPIST ACTIVITY

Therapists will find their activity usefully guided if they consider their every move to have the status of an intervention. In this way, one fully appreciates that no sphere of contact with a family is without diagnostic meaning. There is, for example, no simple socializing that does not simultaneously carry with it information about the performance of that particular family subsystem with the therapist at that moment in the family's interactive life. Minuchin (1974) helpfully categorized interventions into two kinds: those aimed at *accommodation* to the prevailing structures of the family; and *restructuring* moves designed to change family patterns. If therapists were to invoke these rough classifications for each move they made, a great deal of aimless effort would be avoided. The initial self-consciousness in categorizing one's behavior soon gives way to a greater sense of economy and direction, a relief to both the therapist and the family that collectively wishes to experience the therapist as someone in charge of the therapeutic process. Both types of interventions must be used, but intentionally rather than by accident. Here are examples of each type.

A three-generational family, which consisted of several small children, a mother, and the maternal grandmother, arrived for the initial interview. The oldest child, a girl of six, had severe learning difficulties. Within a short time, the therapist had established a tentative map of the family's behavior in a public setting. The maternal grandmother apparently spoke for the family; all the children had reasonable access to her with regard to parental type decisions; meanwhile, the mother sat at the bottom of the hierarchy, with no direct contact with either her children or her mother. A therapist who wished to accommodate to these structural pathways would begin by addressing all communications to the maternal grandmother; instead of contacting the mother directly, the therapist would ask the grandmother to speak to the mother. On the other hand, a therapist who wanted to *restructure* this arrangement would challenge the communicational pathway and speak directly to the mother, perhaps asking her to give the history of the child's difficulty or even information on how the family organized to keep the appointment. The accommodation intervention would allow for one kind of joining, probably an alliance with the grandmother and a temporary estrangement from the mother. The restructuring intervention would promote an alliance with the mother, however uncomfortable for everyone, but would also risk inducing a crisis in the system, perhaps sooner than the therapist would wish. (See Fig. 3-1.)

Like most aspects of structural diagnosis, the content of a therapist's joining moves is less important than alertness to a family's systemic features that are thereby activated. For instance, in the above example, the therapist could simply ask the mother for the names of the children; this behavior would constitute a restructuring move since it opposed the apparent structural preference of the family group.

JOINING AS DIAGNOSIS: EXAMPLES

Here are two examples of an initial diagnostic formulation about family structure made on the basis of joining experiences. The examples illustrate the use of the symbols of structural mapping and the assumption that the therapist's experience of joining the family offers diagnostic information.

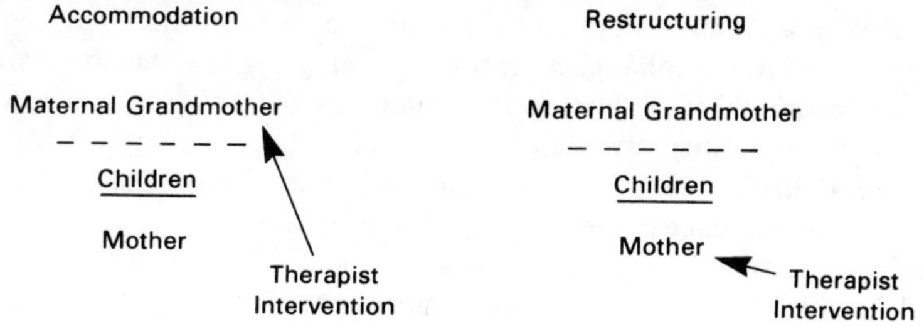

FIGURE 3-1. Two kinds of therapeutic joining into a family group: accommodation and restructuring.

Family A

This family consisted of a father, mother, and their 13-year-old daughter. They were referred because of the daughter's odd behavior in school, including facial grimaces. In addition, she had few friends, and episodes of speaking angrily to her teacher. In the opening minutes of the interview, the therapist, a woman, directed her remarks to all three family members. She noted, however, that both the father and daughter spoke for the mother and that they did this interchangeably and without conflict. The therapist formed a tentative structural map (Fig. 3-2), which showed that access to the family was, so far, through the father–daughter dyad.

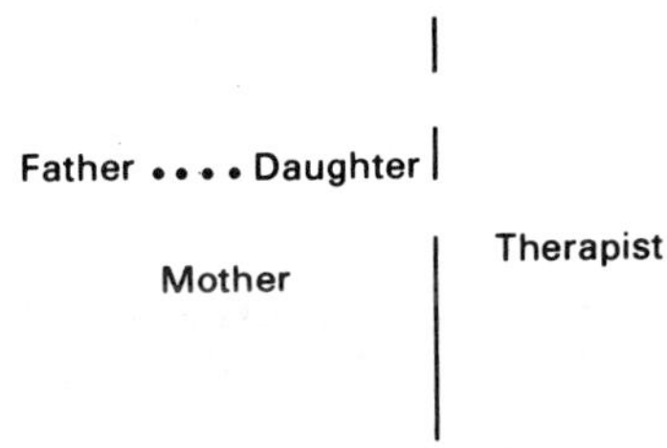

FIGURE 3-2. A tentative structural map of a father–daughter dyad, which apparently has removed the mother from contact with the therapist and which has regulated the therapist's access to the family.

Their relationship was not yet clear, though what did seem apparent was that their activity removed the mother from contact with the therapist.

As the therapist made additional efforts to join the family, she made two more observations. First, the father and daughter knew an enormous amount about each other's lives, including the area of "private thoughts." Second, the mother often prompted either her husband or daughter to tell the therapist about some problem that she, the mother, was having, which was usually a somatic complaint. In this way, the mother reached the therapist, but in compliance with the "speaking-for-her" behavior of the father and daughter. The structural map was then revised to show the father in an enmeshed cross-generational alliance serving as the parental subsystem, itself only diffusely bounded from the mother, who had accepted a lower place in the family hierarchy (see Fig. 3-3). The therapist's access to the family remained regulated by the father–daughter dyad, which, within that format, allowed some contact between the mother and the therapist. The therapist may tentatively conclude that these patterns of

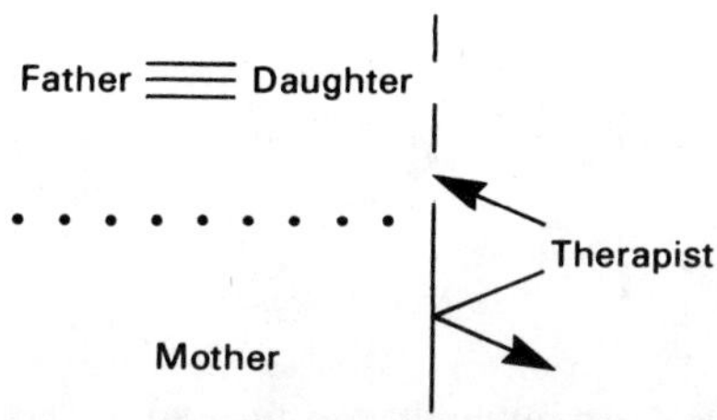

FIGURE 3-3. A revision of the structural map presented in Figure 3-2. The therapist's access to the family continued to be regulated by the father–daughter dyad, but through that dyad, some contact between the mother and the therapist did exist.

alliance and the presence of an inverted executive hierarchy may be a troublesome arrangement, although the rigidity or flexibility of this pattern will not be established until challenged by the active therapist.

Family B

A working-class family was referred because the 16-year-old son is truant from school and in minor troubles with the police. He entered the interview room in a sullen manner, refusing to speak. With him were his two younger brothers, a younger sister, and his parents, who seemed angry and confused. The therapist, a man, noted that the family's initial remarks were all attacks on the eldest son, who continued to sit silently. The therapist tried to join sympathetically with this son (itself a tactical error since it precluded others in the group from finally making such a move). These efforts were routinely interrupted by the father, who did a competent job of describing the son's problems. The wife agreed with her husband. Additional joining moves were made, yielding the following observations: the father encouraged the other children to report on their brother's poor behavior at home and praised them to the therapist when they did so; the wife continued to support her husband; and the sullen son continued to be denied contact with the therapist. The therapist's initial diagnostic map (Fig. 3-4) showed that the therapist could have access to both the parental and the sibling subsystem as long as he complied with the family's coalition against the scapegoated son. This arrangement gave cohesion to the larger family unit, but it removed the oldest son both from the family and from therapeutic contact with the outside world.

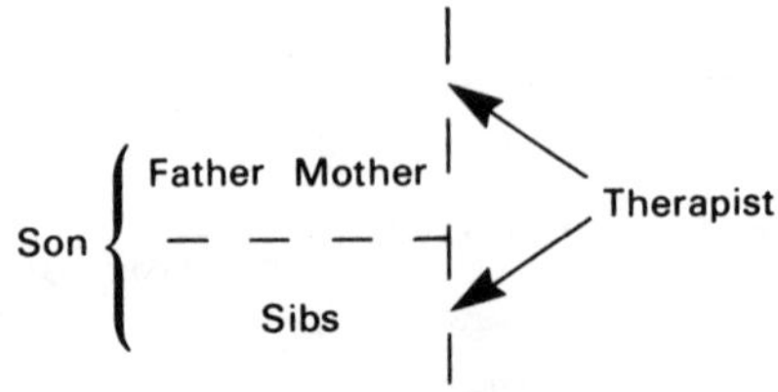

FIGURE 3-4. An initial diagnostic map showing a family in coalition against a scapegoated son. Access to the parental and sibling subsystems in this family existed so long as the therapist complied with the coalition.

SUMMARY

This chapter has presented a view of diagnosis that is explicit in most aspects of structural therapy—that there is no complete systems diagnosis without active efforts by the therapist to alter family functioning and then, most importantly, to make observations of how the family handles such interference. Several styles of therapist activity have been reviewed, and a standard notation for making diagnostic diagrams has been introduced. The task now is to move from these general guidelines to the specific steps one follows in making a distinctively structural diagnosis. That is the work of the next chapter.

Part II

CLINICAL PRACTICE

Chapter 4

Opening Moves: Making a Structural Diagnosis

Here and in the following chapter are described the opening moves a therapist needs to make during the initial contact with a family. Chapters 6, 7, and 8 will then present in greater detail the standard interventions of structural therapy and a discussion of how to consider the resistances to change that make up most of one's therapeutic effort. But before resistance comes the initial contact, a process of joining, diagnosing, and planning that must be relatively successful if a family is to return for a second meeting.

Within the subculture of family therapists, a mystique surrounds the Incredible Initial Interview, a monstrous amalgam of charismatic moves made by Master Therapists (widely publicized in film and book) that dazzle, briefly inspire, and then, too often, simply humble the observer. These impressive performances seem to vanquish forever any hope that one could be as swift or as definitive in one's own therapeutic opening. Everyday therapists admire these great moments in interview history, but secretly despair of having them themselves. Many therapists conclude that great initial interviews belong to the special few and that most ordinary clinicians require greater effort and more time to assess a family thoughtfully. For these reasons, the initial interview is invested with an air of unreality and as such, often seems beyond the grasp of reasonable people. In fact, the initial contact is critical in beginning a successful treatment and offers the clinician an immediate view of nearly all the family's problems and capacities for change. The value of this initial contact can be reasserted when one avoids the confusion between therapist charisma and competent structural therapy techniques. If one allows these technical skills to develop crisply and with force, then the magic of personal charisma becomes less crucial in conducting a competent initial interview. What may seem incredible when others demonstrate it is, as it turns out, quite manageable by us.

Here are the principal goals a therapist hopes to attain in the initial phase with the family:

1. The development of a *structural diagnosis,* including comments on alliances and splits among family members; distinct coalitions; hierarchy problems; boundary problems and properties; and the critical interactional sequences that constitute these structures.
2. The *redefinition of the presenting problem* so that the larger family unit, as well as the symptom-bearing individual, can be intelligently involved in therapeutic change.
3. An assessment of the family's *readiness for change.* This is part of how the therapist redefines the problem and sets treatment goals.
4. The setting of *treatment goals,* done in cooperation with the family so that there is collective agreement about desired outcomes.
5. The *selection of treatment units* and some preliminary planning of *treatment stages,* since not everything will happen at once and not every family member need be involved each step of the way.

ILLUSTRATING DIAGNOSIS

While brief clinical examples are helpful, the more detailed discussions of clinical technique that follow would be better served by a more elaborated case example. The Fletcher family, a composite case, is offered as one illustration of the uses of structural family therapy. Normally when structural therapists begin a new case, they do so without an initially extensive family history; details of the family's life emerge naturally in the pursuit of therapeutic goals. Consistent with that norm, only a brief account of the Fletchers will be given here—no more than what a therapist would receive on the intake sheet. This information would include the presenting problem and the names and relationships of the family members. That is sufficient to begin therapy.

Clinical contact with the Fletchers was precipitated when Irving, Jr., age 17, became involved in a series of school difficulties that caused school authorities to contact his parents. He was doing poorly in his school work, though that had been a somewhat chronic problem. There were more dramatic reasons for the school's concern, however: increased fighting with peers and episodic outbursts of abusive language with several of his male teachers. He was regarded as unpredictable, potentially assaultive, angry, and with only a few redeeming social or scholastic skills. This problem had become more acute during the first semester of his sophomore year at high school, and the school psychologist requested a meeting with Irving and his parents. During the meeting, his parents argued that these behaviors occurred only at school; at home, he was withdrawn and somewhat sullen, but not "bad" or "mean." The mother, however, reluctantly brought up several incidents during which Irving, in the context of a sudden fight with his sisters, set fire to articles of his sister's clothing. His fights with his sister, Judy, were sudden and loud, with no obvious reason for their onset. Mrs. Fletcher usually came to her daughter's aid, thereby becoming involved with Irving's abusive behavior. She did not report these incidents to her husband, seldom expecting him to do anything about them even if he had been aware of their occurrence, and tried to handle them herself. These events had a somewhat bizarre quality to them, and the school counselor, worried that Irving was beginning to show signs of a serious psychological disturbance, referred the family to the local community mental health center. The counselor recommended diagnostic testing for the son, as well as individual diagnostic and treatment interviews. The parents said they were concerned and would follow the referral. Mrs. Fletcher agreed to make the phone call.

Irving was the fifth of six children. He lived at home with his parents and two sisters. Figure 4-1 presents the family composition. Throughout the book, we will follow this family during the course of its treatment.

The beginning structural family therapist is now prepared with intake information, some symbols of a structural diagnosis, and some assumptions about the relationship of joining a family to a diagnosis of its problems. Now the opening moves of a structural approach to family therapy may begin. In the chapters that follow, these initial moves are described, as are the intervention strategies that are most characteristic of a structural approach. The inevitable resistances and failures that follow the

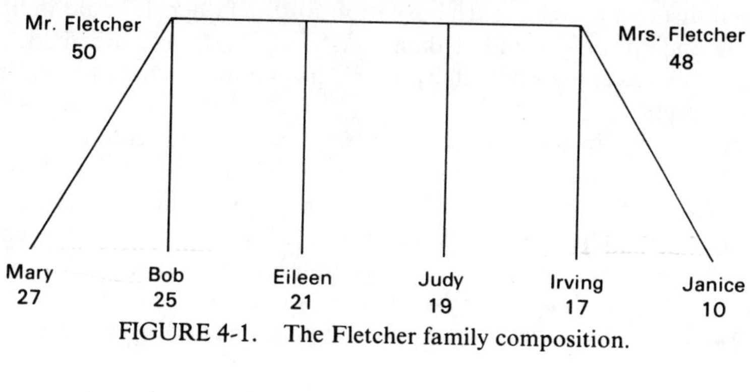

FIGURE 4-1. The Fletcher family composition.

initial phase of treatment will be given special attention, since so much of effective psychotherapy is knowing how to go ahead when all the theoretically correct moves have not helped the family.

THE STRUCTURAL DIAGNOSIS

A structural diagnosis is a series of statements about (1) the alliances and coalitions within the family; (2) the boundary properties of the total family and its subsystems; (3) the hierarchical distribution of executive power; and (4) the key interactional behaviors that make up these abstracted structures and give experiential meaning to them. Above all, a structural diagnosis is a hypothesis about the systemic interaction between the total family context and the symptomatic behaviors of the individual members. All of these features become evident in the initial contact with the Fletchers.

When the Fletcher family arrived for its initial interview, all family members were present except for Bob, the oldest son. The focus was on Irving, and it would be the task of the therapist, a man in his early thirties, to conduct the interview in such a way that Irving's peculiar behaviors might be understood as sensible responses to strains within the larger family unit. In this way, matters of individual "character" become behavior-in-context.

The therapist, who allowed the family to precede him into the interview room, noted something curious about the seating arrangement (see Fig. 4-2): the father's position left him partially isolated, although whether he was at the head or at the end of the family circle was unclear. The therapist noted that the two men, the father and Irving, were separated from each other by the women and that the mother was flanked by the two daughters living at home. This seating forced the therapist to enter by sitting next to the father; the meaning of the father's place was uncertain. It could indicate a pattern of true isolation for the father. It could indicate that he and Mary, the oldest daughter, were the family members who customarily accepted contact by outsiders. Or it could be an entirely random event.

After some introductions and a moment of social contact with all family members (barely achieved with Irving, who slumped sullenly in his chair), the therapist asked what problem brought them to the clinic and how he might help. Mrs. Fletcher responded quickly and competently, offering a summary of the school's complaint and a brief comment on Irving's misbehavior at home. Near the end of her reply, the two daughters living at home completed some of her sentences and added a few criticisms

Father

Therapist — Janice (10)

Mary (27) — Mother

Eileen (21) — Judy (19)

Irving (17)

FIGURE 4-2. The seating arrangement of the Fletcher family members during the family's initial interview.

of their own. Mr. Fletcher then reaffirmed the family's concern, speaking as a somewhat formal representative of all present. He emphasized their determination to help Irving and briefly agreed with his wife's synopsis. Throughout this, Irving was silent; his head was lowered and his attitude a mixture of defiance and shame. He appealed to no one, nor were there any sympathetic offers of support. Thus, the opening moments concluded.

This is an important punctuation. The family seems united in criticism of the son and, as a unit, in temporary systems equilibrium. It is a perfect point in time for the therapist, as a force outside the system, to explore ways in which the family might change. Based on the opening moments, he can form a very tentative diagnostic map (Fig. 4-3) about alliances among family members: Mrs. Fletcher and the daughters, themselves rather closely joined, seem in coalition against the patient. The ties between the father and son are not yet clear, so they are presented as diffusely present. Figure 4-3 also gives visual representation to the experience of these opening moments—namely, that the father and son do not seem connected in any positive way to each other or to other family members. The therapist also notes that the initial discussion constitutes an interactional sequence that may reappear later:

1. The mother begins listing critical concerns about the son.
2. She is joined by the daughters.
3. They are joined by the father.
4. This coalition is not challenged by the son.

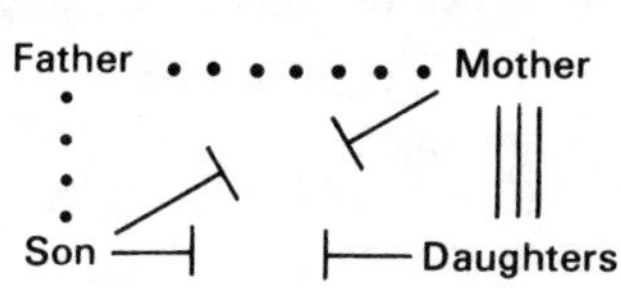

FIGURE 4-3. Tentative diagnostic map of Fletcher family alliances.

One further bit of information is available: the father apparently is *not* the head of the family circle, but brings up the end and in that way becomes included. These musings and the diagnostic map may be used as a guide, but must be considered very tentative.

The therapist is now faced with several options. The least useful of these is to say nothing, perhaps hoping his silence will slow the scapegoating process. This would be a poor response to a family looking for help. But the other options for response must be viewed carefully, since the therapist does not wish, as a result of error, to become the third isolated man in this group. The problem and possible therapist responses are presented in Table 4-1. The structural therapist attempts to activate a new sequence of behavior by first acknowledging the obvious—that Irving is silent in the face of attack—and then locating the responsibility for moving ahead as entirely the family's. The family must respond to this silence, which the therapist suggests, although he remains noncommittal about who should make the contact with Irving. This is in clear contrast to other possible therapist behaviors, such as (1) attributing to Irving an internal feeling ("You must be really upset") or (2) emphasizing to Irving the *therapist's* concern and neutrality. These efforts, though intended to console the patient and resist the scapegoating process, are errors. They prevent a therapist from seeing who in the family might break out of the attacking coalition to help Irving, and, implicitly, they criticize the family, suggesting that only the therapist is sympathetic.

The options may be further refined if one recalls that a therapist's interventions may be of two kinds—accommodating or restructuring. The therapist could either respect the apparent structure or challenge it by confronting the problems of alliance or of hierarchy. Of the three possible remarks presented in Table 4-2, the last one is the most daring and the most likely to fail, especially so early in an interview; it presumes there is a hierarchical dysfunction and exposes this presumption by asking the

Table 4-1
POSSIBLE THERAPIST RESPONSES TO THE SCAPEGOATING PROBLEM IN THE FLETCHER FAMILY

Problem	Structural Therapist	Other Therapist
A system stuck with the completion of a scapegoating sequence	"Only Irving has said nothing so far. Who can get his side of the story?"	"Irving, you must be really upset by all this." *OR* "Irving, *I* am really interested in your side of this."

Table 4-2
POSSIBLE THERAPIST INTERVENTIONS IN FLETCHER FAMILY

Accommodation	Alliance Restructuring	Hierarchy Restructuring
"Mrs. Fletcher, I wonder if you could get Irving's side of the story?"	"Mr. Fletcher, perhaps you and Irving could discuss his side of the story."	"Mr. Fletcher, perhaps you could get your wife to find out more about her son's view of this matter."

father to direct the mother. Nonetheless, it may become a desirable choice if the other moves fail.

The therapist, in fact, made his first intentional *restructuring* intervention, asking the father to engage his son:

	INTERVIEW	COMMENTARY
Therapist:	Mr. Fletcher, perhaps you and Irving could discuss his side of the story.	This is a move to restructure the alliance between father and son. It rests on an initial and untested structural diagnosis.
Father:	I don't think he will say. . . .	The father resists the therapist, and his wife tries to reassert her leadership of sequences.
Mother:	(Interrupting) Won't say a word of explanation or even of apology to me or the. . . .	
Therapist:	(Interrupting) But wait a minute, your husband was just beginning his effort, and Irving might . . . he was . . . please, go ahead and finish, Mr. Fletcher.	The therapist continues his intervention by blocking the mother and suggesting that the test has not yet failed.
Father:	Well, Irving. What's this about what your mother says, that you set these fires, burning your sister's shirts and stuff and all.	Father tries again, but under cover of his wife's complaints, thereby resisting the therapist and avoiding alliance with the son.
Irving:	(Remains silent.)	
Therapist:	That's a good beginning, and it lets your wife know you really share her concern. But what about moving beyond that for just a minute and really helping your son say his piece. Just to you.	The therapist still continues, calling it a "good beginning," but redirecting father to son.

Father:	I don't know . . . is there something you can tell me? I would listen, no punishments for what you say or anything like that. Did they do something or what?	Father's response indicates hope for the intervention.
Irving:	They bug me, always full of . . . always snotty and against me.	The content of this exchange is unimportant. What matters is that the son and father are joined together, however briefly, without the mother's intrusion.
Father:	Yeah, but I mean what did they. . . .	
Irving:	Just everything, all . . . like last night. . . .	

This brief exchange teaches three things. First, it shows the active persistence required of a therapist and the need to continue an intervention until it succeeds or has definitely failed at that time. Too frequently, therapists begin something and then quickly relinquish the effort, a resignation that may suggest to the family that no real change is expected by the therapist. Secondly, one is always alert to signs of flexibility in family alliances; here, the father and son do demonstrate an ability to get together, and the mother exhibits an ability to accept that. Finally, there is some additional evidence for the original diagnostic impression that the mother tends to take over the initiation of behavioral sequences.

DATA FOR A STRUCTURAL DIAGNOSIS

Thus engaged, the therapist can continue to gather diagnostic information. But what constitutes information for a structural therapist? There are four customary sources of data available:

1. The data of historical report
2. The data of directed behavior: enacting family problems
3. The data of natural behavior
4. The data of the family's response to the therapist's efforts to join and change them

In pursuit of this information, the therapist and family will engage in a variety of behaviors, some spontaneous and some evoked by the therapist. A consideration of each of these sources of data shows several principles of the structural approach.

The Data of Historical Report

Structural therapists usually consider this the least useful source of information about family functioning. It is often unreliable, colored by the imperfect recall of whoever tells the story, and usually replete with tempting bits of information about the intrapsychic life of the patient. Inexperienced therapists often succumb to temptation and soon find themselves chasing down the "roots" of the problem in some *cul-de-sac* of ancient instinctual clashes when the patient was three years old. (The problems of discussing psychological content were discussed in Chapter 1.) Structuralists have argued that these stories are not only incapable of verification (and hence, poor sources of data for any scientific theory), but they paralyze change with the implicit hopelessness of a linear model. Families, for example, frequently invoke linear causality in such a way that change is difficult to imagine, since the original insult cannot be undone. If you are crazy at the age of 18 because you were dropped on your head at age two, or frightened by an animal when you were five (as some famous people were), then what's to be done? Although initially the psychological content may be exciting and the mystery of the missing links compelling to one's linear longings, both the family and therapist may soon find themselves burdened by some rather ominous conclusions and without much spirit for the present-day fray. This is the usual argument against history as diagnostically useful data.

This argument is also an overstatement, one best understood with reference to the historical content within which structural family therapy developed. Eager to avoid notions of linear causality, the structuralists once assiduously avoided all intrapsychic material—memories, dreams, reflections, and feelings—and consequently needed to minimize history, inasmuch as it was these inner events that populated the past. In short, it was not so much the past itself that was suspect, but the implicit linearity and the inevitable distortions of recall that made stories of the past poor data for the *circular* paradigm of behavior. Hence, history as "reported fact" was discarded, though history as "contemporary experience"—that is, the telling about the family past as a here-and-now behavior exchange among family members—could be retained as a "process" event. Now that the structural viewpoint is less embattled, there is less need for such a dogmatic dismissal of a family's historical development. For example, it helps the therapist to know that a husband's apparent indifference to his wife is, with regard to his family-of-origin, an act of loyalty since his family had historically disapproved of his wife. No matter how perceptively the structural therapist analyzes contemporary behavior sequences of this family, the husband's behavior will remain a puzzle. It is not necessary to impute unconscious loyalties to the husband or to posit any other intrapsychic event. It is, however, necessary to recognize that, historically, over time, the husband spontaneously belonged to two contexts, his family-of-origin and his own nuclear family. In this way, history becomes meaningful data in viewing a contemporary, contextual behavior—the husband's immobility and indifference toward his wife.

The Data of Directed Behavior

This is a highly preferred source of data about family experience. What happens in the initial interview, both spontaneously and in response to the therapist, offers for observation those interactional behaviors that presumably make up the structures of family life. Structural therapy emphasizes observations of behavior-in-context and in the here and now, rather than reports about behavior in the past. While the content of the family's story fills the air space, the therapist is ignoring that, preferring instead to observe the interactive process that is the medium for conveying any particular message. But what precisely does one observe?

A Note on Seeing Structure

It's simple enough to advise one to observe the "family at work." But what does one look for? Among thousands of possibilities, which bits of behavior does the therapist select and, in the very act of selection, arbitrarily award to them the status of data? The intention of any theory is to bias observations so that the underlying premises are supported, while the ability to disprove the secondary hypotheses derived from those premises is retained. So, for example, the observing therapist is not expected to test the grand assumptions of structural theory, but rather to ask if there is information as to *which* alliances seem most open and which seem most concealed, which subunits are well bounded and which are poorly bounded, and so forth. The therapist puts on the structural "spectacles" in order to see something in family life other than psychological content and linear developments. Whether or not this view of matters is correct or even the most helpful perspective is a debate on another level. While in the thick of an initial structural interview, the therapist simply assumes the bias and searches for behaviors relevant to it. For example, the therapist may attend to who speaks to whom, who looks to whom for support, and who opposes whom, rather than note the content of what is being said. The therapist looks for who sits with whom, listens to reports of who affiliates with whom at home, and listens to how decisions are made, which indicates something about power and hierarchies. The therapist notes how well or poorly family members seem to know the important details of each other's lives, knowledge that may suggest how enmeshed or disengaged is the family or its subunits. In brief, the therapist "observes," that is, collects and stores those transactional events that are relevant to a description of family structure. For example, consider this exchange between members of the Fletcher family:

Mother: Of course, my own mother tells me Irving has always been a bit, a little . . . well, since he was three and fell off that swing.

Judy: And grandmother is close to it so . . . see, she would know what mother and I are saying. Besides, when Irving gets into my clothes, well it's just weird. I think he's just a retard and a faggot and. . . .

Eileen: But we all used to trade clothes. Not defending Irving, but Mary and I traded, and you and I traded. And we didn't ask.

Mary: But we're women. I mean this is just too strange with him. And when he was little, he had that doll he wouldn't let go of. That little . . . couldn't tell if it was a boy or girl doll, but, like after his accident, he would cry and stuff and remember and all.

Irving: That was your goddamn doll. I never had one. (Angrily) And I never touched your clothes, so why take their side?

Mother: Your sisters are just telling the truth. That's why we are here—to tell the truth, 'cause you have to stop, and if you have funny feelings about yourself, then tell the doctor.

Father: Yeah, but slow down a bit. He probably did . . . I mean. . . .

Mother: (Interrupting) No! He should say right now, right away if he's got funny ideas, because he's got to stop this stuff with the girls. I won't stand for it anymore.

There is a good deal in this exchange to arouse questions about Irving's sexual identity and about the onset of such problems. Broad hints are offered that he is too interested in "girls' things" and that his "accident" at age three is the beginning of a troubled developmental history. This may be of interest to a therapist oriented to psychological content, but the structural therapist, in order to stay on track, should choose instead to note the following: (1) The mother seems closely joined with her daughters, who themselves apparently constitute a strong subunit of sisters; (2) the maternal grandmother is a considerable force in the family and especially present in her daughter's life, evidently more so than is Mr. Fletcher; this suggests three generations of mother–daughter closeness, although there is no reason yet to label it as enmeshment; and (3) neither father nor Irving is able to make a significant impact on this well-bounded subsystem of women.

The structural therapist must not only learn to make new observations, ones different than those made from a psychodynamic orientation, but must also be responsible for encouraging an interactive process that will provide the raw behaviors of family routine. The therapist can do this in several ways: (1) by giving neutral directions that encourage an interactive process; (2) by changing the interview context itself; and (3) by giving restructuring directions.

	NEUTRAL DIRECTIONS	COMMENTARY
Therapist:	Now that Mr. Fletcher and Irving have talked, maybe you all can talk over what you have heard. It would help to hear the family discuss all this.	This is an open and general invitation, carefully directed at no particular family member.
Mother:	What do you want?	Again, the mother leads, mounting some resistance. The therapist continues in an accommodating way, accepting the mother's leadership, but using her to help begin the family interactions he needs to observe.
Therapist:	For the whole family to discuss this.	
Mother:	I already know what Judy thinks.	
Therapist:	So perhaps you can start her and the others discussing it.	

The intention of these neutral directions is to evoke activity, feeling, and discussion among the family members about the presenting problem. Therapists need to "track" (Minuchin's phrase) the content, probing carefully to recover the details of family routine, of exactly what commonplace exchanges and daily activities characterize this particular family. Without evidence of actual behavioral exchanges, it is impossible to make deductions about structural issues. When such accounts and discussions have begun, the therapist should assume the status of a visiting anthropologist, peering over the perimeter of the family-unit-boundary into the workings of this small society, making mental notes about the family's way of conducting business. As mentioned earlier, the therapist, now an observer, is looking for information about alliances, coalitions, hierarchies, boundary attributes, and repetitive, circular sequences of behavior, all of which may help the therapist to understand the particular symptomatic behavior of the index patient. During this period, comments to the therapist should be redirected, in a neutral and structurally accommodating way, to the family as a whole. The emphasis is now on observing the family at work.

A second way of eliciting behavioral activity is to alter the largest parameters of the context within which the interview is being conducted. This means to change the actual groupings of the people present and is in accord with a fundamental principle of systems theory; that is, one alters the larger context as one requires its component parts to behave differently. The therapist may alter the context in (1) brief ways, such as inviting two members of the family to talk with each other while the others remain as observers, or in (2) broad ways, such as meeting for longer periods of time with subunits of the family, temporarily excluding from the interview room and process the rest of the family.

	CONTEXT DIRECTIONS	COMMENTARY
Therapist:	I've noticed that Irving's brother, Bob, is not here, and I think, well, that's hard to be surrounded only by sisters. I think something would be learned if the girls waited outside. And they have been helpful, and I'll see you later. Would you mind waiting outside for a while now? (Gestures to the daughters.)	The therapist attempts to give a positive frame for his request. His move is a direct intervention against the strong subsystem of women. His intent is to see if a change in interpersonal context will allow the father and Irving to behave differently, without knowing *what* the difference might be. This direction is not immediately successful, and why it fails is quite instructive, suggesting the presence of a *sequence* that elicits Irving's angry behavior. Here, note that the therapist achieves partial success only after some effort and only after Irving and Judy have entered into their usual fight, one of the problems that prompted the referral.
Judy:	I'd rather be with them than with this creep. (To the mother) Is that O.K. with you?	
Mother:	Maybe the older girls could leave, but Judy is the one who is most involved here.	
Therapist:	So she should stay with you? Not her sisters?	
Judy:	But this doesn't involve me. It's his crazy stuff.	
Mother:	No. But you know more and that would help the doctor. I mean, it *is* Irving, but you should tell what you know.	
Irving:	Sure, stay and lie as usual. And I'll tell what a tramp you are.	
Judy:	You're crazy. You don't believe that (looking at the mother)? I'm not moving.	
Mother:	(Speaking to son) You can't speak to her like that! (Looking at Judy) I know you're not doing anything wrong, so you can stay right here.	
Therapist:	Since Judy can't leave, would you two go on out? (Gesturing to Mary and Eileen, who leave.)	Finally, the two older daughters do leave, showing their greater autonomy. The therapist will now observe how Irving behaves in this smaller unit.

This effort to change the context seems neutral enough. It is simply a division of the siblings according to sex and a removal of the son from his surrounding sisters in an effort to elicit something other than his silence or anger. The response of the family, however, suggests that there is nothing neutral about the therapist's request. On the contrary, a particular fight sequence follows. Indeed, many requests for a change of context may elicit such responses, and while the therapist's direction should not be considered a failure, attention should be paid to how, in this particular situation, the direction is not entirely effective. In this way, new information is gained about the subsystems and alliances in the family.

In addition to neutral directions and context directions, the therapist may elicit data about family behavior by offering restructuring interventions. This is a variation of altering the wider context. It avoids any effort to be neutral but instead frankly directs some members of the family to form, briefly and artificially, a new context, a restructured grouping that will permit new behavior and tell the therapist how flexibly or rigidly the family can move into improved patterns of interaction.

	RESTRUCTURING DIRECTIONS	COMMENTARY
Therapist:	Now, Mr. Fletcher. I would like you and your wife to trade seats so that you can sit right next to Irving while you two men talk all this over. And Mrs. Fletcher, I want you to sit here next to me, relax a bit, and let your husband take care of things. (He gestures for them to stand up.)	Regardless of what follows, the therapist feels encouraged that the parents will shift the alliances to the son, although the mother is clearly a bit reluctant. The therapist tries to suggest (1) that there are two men in the room who need to be linked; (2) that the mother has had too great a burden; and (3) that she can trust her husband to handle the son. It now remains for the therapist to observe how people behave in this new, restructured context. The emergence of new and less charged behaviors will be encouraging, while the persistence of old behaviors, in spite of the context change, will point to some pathological rigidity of the system.
Mother:	You mean now?	
Therapist:	Yeah. (The therapist is now standing.)	
Mother:	If it will help. (She stands.)	
Father:	I don't know. . . . (He moves to wife's chair.)	
Therapist:	Just for a few minutes, till we get this thing going.	

The Data of Natural Behavior

Another source of data based on the actual interview experience comes from observing apparently spontaneous behaviors among family members. "Apparently" is a necessary qualifier, since most behavior occurs (1) in the context of contemporary exchanges with others and (2) at a certain point in the sequence that makes up one of these exchanges. Minuchin and Fishman (1981) noted that such spontaneous events are excellent moments for intervention, since the therapist can highlight and intensify this "nonevent" into a revealing and symptomatic transaction that compels the family to appreciate the pervasiveness of certain patterns of living. There are, of course, truly novel and original behaviors that can move the system to a new and different level of organization. With that exception (and with a good deal of time allotted in order to judge a behavior), most of the family's activity remains context bound. To speak of "spontaneous" events is simply to note that things happen quite beyond the intended direction of the therapist or beyond any apparent instigation from a family member. There is no readily discernible mover, or if there is one, the sequence of behaviors thus begun seems to bear little relevance to the mainstream of family movement.

For example, during the second half of the interview, the therapist has the father and mother talking together and is trying to assess the possibility of moving them closer together in parenting tasks. While they are chatting about Irving, the following exchange occurs among the older children (Mary and Eileen have returned to the room):

	SPONTANEOUS EXCHANGES	COMMENTARY
Judy:	(Speaking to Mary in a whisper) Is that a new blouse?	This exchange among the older children occurs off-stage and seems disruptive to the therapist's effort to allow the parents a separate space. The sponanteity of the exchange may, however, suggest at least two hypotheses: (1) that a family rule has evolved to prohibit the parents from forming an effective subunit, in which case, they must be interrupted; or (2) that the actual arrangement of who speaks to whom and in what order constitutes a *sequence* with psychological and systemic integrity. Such sequences are important codes about the family's structure. This particular sequence is similar to one reported earlier and is commented on below.
Mary:	It's Eileen's. She just got it and let me wear it today.	
Judy:	It's neat. Could I wear. . . .	
Mother:	(Speaking directly to Judy) Please don't interrupt, dear. You need to hear this as well as me.	
Irving:	(Speaking to Judy) You wouldn't look good in it anyway.	

The Data of the Family's Response to the Therapist

How the family accommodates to or resists the therapist tells a great deal about their internal structural map. These are the data that emerge when joining experiences are viewed as one type of diagnostic data. The preceding chapter on joining as diagnosis offers some examples. In the case of the Fletcher family, the therapist learns several things as he maneuvers for entrance and power within the family. First, Mrs. Fletcher remains the principal gatekeeper when the entire family is present; the effective passing of information across the family-unit-boundary is most easily done by accommodating to this rule. Second, any effort to make an alliance with Irving, the beleaguered son, only firms up the remaining family members into a coalition that excludes Irving. Third, in meeting with subunits of the family, the therapist discovers a relatively easy access to the group of daughters; they chat freely among themselves and accept the therapist's remarks in a confident and balanced manner. Conversely, in spending a few minutes alone with the father and Irving, the therapist senses little connection between them and, as with any disengaged dyad, has to work very hard to elicit any interest, on either of their parts, in forming a working coalition. They tend to agree with the therapist at all times and offer no collective resistance or moderation of the therapist's inputs.

THE INITIAL STRUCTURAL DIAGNOSIS

Using these four sources of data (history, the interview experience, spontaneous events, and the impact of the therapist-as-joiner), a series of initial diagnostic statements can be made. These are tentative in the sense that they are hypotheses to be tested in subsequent interviews. They are not tentative, however, as the guidelines for immediate therapist activity directed toward helping the family deal with its problem. Here are the parts that make up a structural diagnostic statement.

Alliances and Splits

Throughout the initial interview with the Fletchers, considerable information emerges about the mother's family-of-origin and her continued close ties with her mother and her younger sister. There is correspondingly little evidence of the father's tie to anyone. Figures 4-4 and 4-5 present diagrams of the alliance structure within the Fletchers' extended nuclear family. These diagrams summarize an impression that the mother is overly close to her mother and her sister and, a generation

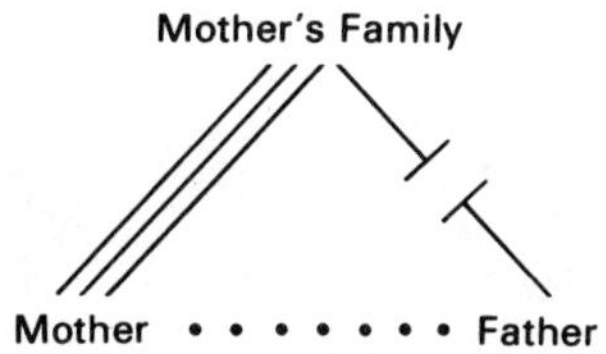

FIGURE 4-4. The Fletchers' extended family.

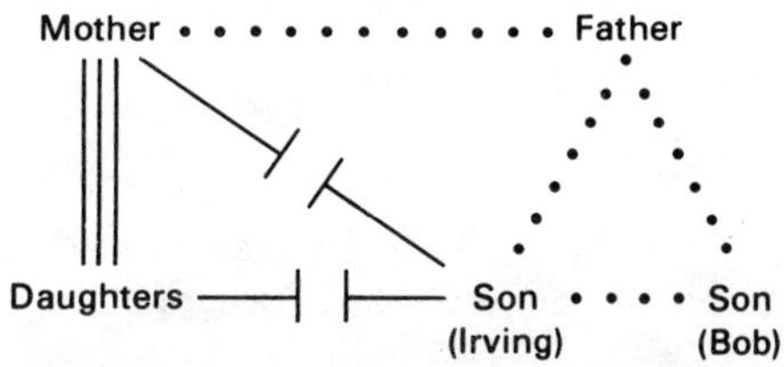

FIGURE 4-5. The Fletchers' nuclear family.

down, to her own daughters, both those living at home and those living away. To this extent, she is removed from her husband who himself seems without close ties, either within the family or outside it. Next, the son is depicted as relatively isolated in the family through his diffuse tie with the father and his hostile relationship with his sisters. Finally, the other son, Bob, is not only absent from this interview, but so seldom mentioned as to confirm a growing conviction that the men in this family are isolated and without a strong subsystem of their own.

Coalitions

In many groups and in all triangular arrangements, there is a natural tendency to form coalitions, a systemic movement not in itself necessarily bad. Caplow (1968) has argued that all triangles, for example, are constantly in a revolving process of forming coalitions of two against one. When these coalitions become stuck and rigid, pathological consequences may result, especially for the person excluded from the coalition. In the case of the Fletcher family, an alarming capacity to form just such a coalition of all its members against Irving is apparent. There are two rather faint exceptions to this rule. First, the father seems a bit reluctant to join in attacking his son, and one suspects he does so as his only way of appearing to be still in the family in a position of power. Second, the older sisters seem to have little investment in the designation of Irving as troublemaker. They seem preoccupied with him only when the parents are present.

Hierarchy Problems

The interview experience itself reveals a disturbance in the hierarchical distribution of executive power. The mother and Judy act like the effective parents to Irving and Janice, the youngest daughter, while the father is somewhat excluded. (See Fig. 4-6.)

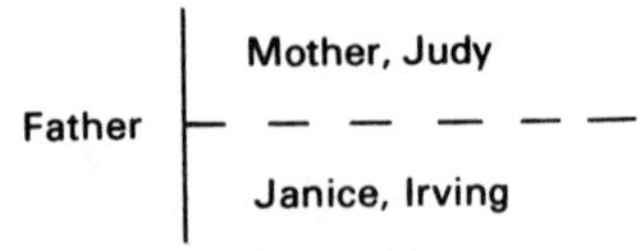

FIGURE 4-6. Diagram of hierarchical distribution of executive power in the Fletcher family.

Boundary Properties

Several statements can be made about boundary operations in the Fletcher family. The family as a whole, for example, does let in and send information to an outsider, as long as the outsider complies with the rule that the mother is initially to manage the joining activity. Within the family, the boundary issues are not so encouraging. For example, the boundary between the mother and her nuclear family is diffuse, permitting an overregulation of the nuclear family by the influence of the maternal grandmother. On the other hand, the boundary *around* the women in the family is relatively closed to new members or new ideas. This closed boundary is apparent within the nuclear family and in all the female members across three generations. (See Fig. 4-7.) The comparable boundary that might be drawn around the subunit of men, the father and the two sons, is so diffuse as to afford them no articulated identity at all. (See Fig. 4-8.) It can also be observed that when parenting operations do occur (regardless of who becomes a member of the parenting unit), the boundary between the children and the parental subunit seems open and adaptive.

Critical Sequences

The analysis of transactional sequences as a therapeutic tactic will be discussed in Chapter 6. The recognition of such sequences is, however, an

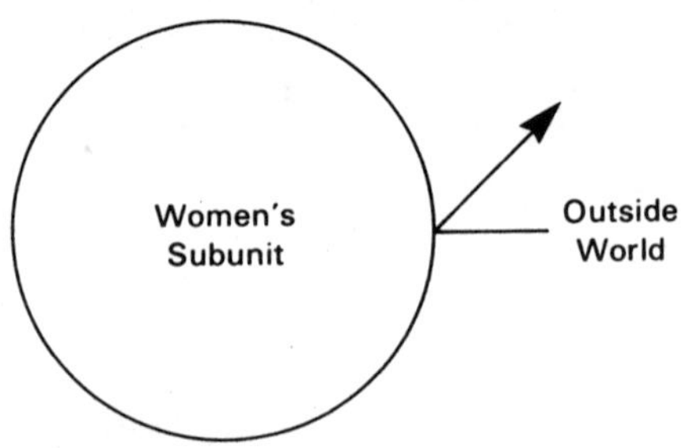

FIGURE 4-7. Boundary operations in the Fletcher family: the female subunit.

important part of a structural diagnosis. One particular sequence in the initial interview is crucial to a major notion about what is going on in this family. This is the sequence noted earlier (p. 67), and in an expanded discussion, presents the following points:

1. The rigid and closed unit boundary around the women momentarily relaxes, as when the therapist attempts to have the daughters separate from the others (or when, in a later sequence, Judy starts a whispered conversation with those sisters living away from home). During these moments, Judy tries to move away from the mother and into alliance with her older sisters. If successful and repeated, this move would restructure the larger group of women into two smaller groups—one composed of older daughters seeking more autonomy and a second group consisting of the mother and the women in her family-of-origin.
2. But this tentative move activates a quick counterresponse from the mother, who on both occasions insists that Judy stay with her. In the first occurrence, she does not want Judy to leave the room with her older sisters. Later, she prevents Judy from talking with the older girls. The quickness of the mother's move is typical of an overly close alliance or enmeshment.
3. Irving then enters the action and attacks Judy, threatening to tell the others that she is a "tramp." (In a later sequence, he tells Judy she wouldn't look attractive in the blouse of Mary's that she admires.)
4. Judy responds by returning the attack and thus returning to her mother's side. The mother now moves to defend Judy from Irving, thereby strengthening the tie between herself and her daughter.
5. A strong subunit boundary is restored (around the women) and the entire system returns to a homeostatic plateau. Part of this balance requires the absence of Mr. Fletcher who, indeed, is noticeably excluded in this sequence.

This is an extended description of a critical sequence, one that occurs several times in the interview and that therefore attracts the attention of the therapist. He follows this up with some questions about Irving's misbehavior at home and finds, with great particulars, the same sequence, although at home the nature of Irving's attack on the girls takes the form of fire-setting or obscene language. A briefer summary of the sequence would look like this:

1. A subunit boundary (around Judy and the mother) is relaxed; Judy moves toward the outside.
2. The mother quickly counters, reclaiming Judy's alliance.
3. Irving attacks Judy.
4. Judy and the mother now team up to defend against the attack.

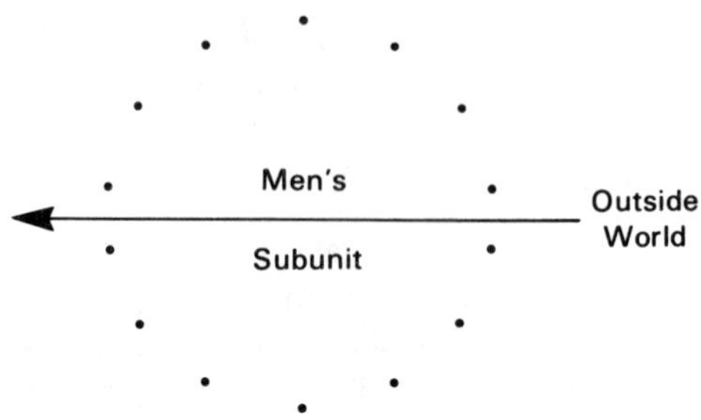

FIGURE 4-8. Boundary operations in the Fletcher family: the male subunit.

5. Equilibrium is restored, and a new sequence may now begin. This analysis prompts a revision of the earlier impression that all the women were equally included in the subunit of women. Clearly, the two older girls who are living away from home have a lesser role and show signs of forming their own autonomous unit.

A DIAGNOSTIC SUMMARY

At this point, an initial diagnostic impression emerges, one that attempts to relate the presenting problem of an individual member to larger issues within the family system. Based only on the experiential data of the first interview and some brief historical report, the diagnosis can be reported in two ways—in diagram form and, more fully, in a short statement.

Structural Diagram

In the preceding diagrams of alliances, hierarchies, and boundaries within the Fletcher family, the therapist must decide which of these structures needs the most diagnostic emphasis. This choice reflects the therapist's judgment about where the greatest disturbance lies. Diagrams may show all sectors of family structure, but generally one principal direction of this initial diagnosis becomes the main diagram. For the Fletchers, the issues of alliance and, secondarily, the subgroupings thereby implied seem more important than whatever hierarchical imbalances may be present. An extended diagram of the alliance structure is shown in Figure 4-9. This diagram summarizes some diagnostic information. The mother is clearly the recipient of both normal and overly close ties with other female members of the family, including her extended family. She is

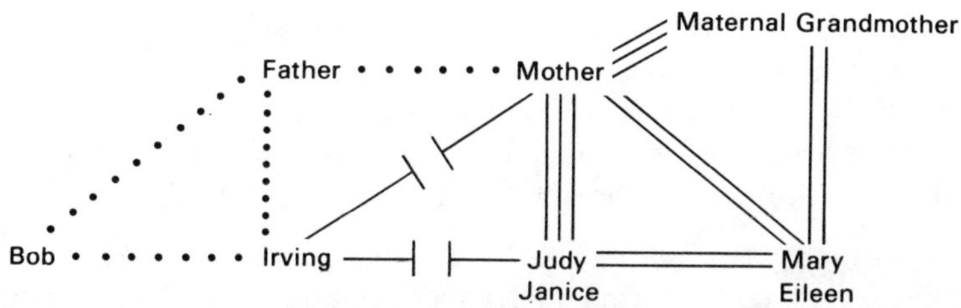

FIGURE 4-9. An extended diagram of the alliance structure in the Fletcher family.

only diffusely or hostilely related to the men. Conversely, alliances among the men are either diffuse or unknown, as with Bob, the older brother. Irving receives active contact with the women in the form of attack and fighting. He appears without any strong positive alliances. This is also true of Mr. Fletcher.

A Structural Statement

The following statements have the status of hypotheses, useful in guiding subsequent interventions, but subject to revision as new information emerges. The hypotheses include the following:

1. The mother has been a member of enmeshed subunits, first with her own mother and later with her daughters, especially Judy.
2. Over time, a structural schism has developed in the family. The women have formed an apparently well-bounded, though somewhat enmeshed, subunit, while the men have generally been disengaged from each other as well as from the family as a whole.
3. This homeostatic norm is sometimes coincidental with the normal life-cycle stage when a family helps the teenage children leave home. During such a coincidence, trouble may develop.
4. There is an inappropriate parenting subsystem composed of the mother and Judy, with the father very much on the periphery.
5. Both the homeostasis of the larger family unit and the balance of the parenting unit are threatened whenever Judy attempts to move outside these boundaries and join the sibling group of sisters living away from home.
6. A preliminary analysis of Irving's symptoms shows them to occur in a critical sequence that involves exchanges between himself, his mother, and Judy. His symptomatic behavior, including his difficulty with male teachers, is part of a systems phenomena that restores

equilibrium by reinvolving Judy with the mother; ironically provides some contact, however conflicted, between the men and the women; establishes the need for more central fathering; and provides the father with at least temporary membership in the parenting subsystem on those occasions when he joins the family in scapegoating his son.

In summary, within the context of a deep schism dividing the male from the female family members, Irving's symptoms reflect his absence of core membership in a firmly identified male subunit, complete with the male models needed in adolescence, and his unwitting role in helping his mother reaffirm both the tight boundaries of the women's subunit and her place within it. Without the reinforcement of these symptomatic behaviors, Judy might be freed to move away from her mother and eventually away from home, as her older sisters have done. This would leave the mother more available to possible connections with her husband. Or, stated from the husband's position, if he were more forcefully to initiate behaviors that would help his children differentiate from the larger family unit by joining their appropriate subunits, then he would be positioned to have more contact with his wife. The son's symptoms and family response to them form behavioral sequences that prevent this from happening.

Summary

The extended statement just made and the diagram (Fig. 4-9) before it comprise the hypotheses of a structural diagnosis. There is primary emphasis on the properties of systemic functioning (boundaries, alliances, sequences, etc.), though this does not prevent reference to the psychological phenomena traditionally associated with the development of individual lives within the larger family group. For example, having made statements about subunit properties, one can further add that boys usually profit, especially during adolescence, from benevolent associations with interested fathers. Similarly, after noting that Irving's symptoms provide an opportunity for Mr. and Mrs. Fletcher to demonstrate publicly that they are unified as parents, one can then register some doubt about their private motivations for being closer as marital partners. To make a structural diagnostic statement is to say something about the way people are positioned for contact, with each other and with other subsystems. It does not necessarily prevent one from making further assumptions about those events one cannot observe, such as inner wishes and feelings. This statement simply makes such assumptions inessential in drawing up plans about what to do. A structural diagnosis should tell the therapist about the relational position of each subunit within the larger system and the readiness of these units to assume new, altered states of contact with each other. Where any particular subunit is in a poor "systems position," there is a correspondingly reduced possibility for healthy contact. One may, for example, speak of Mr. and Mrs. Fletcher's structural positions as ones with minimal possibilities for contact with each other. To change Mr. Fletcher's position—which would happen, for example, if he were brought into closer proximity to his son—would change his overall systems position. This, in theory, increases his possibility for contact with his wife, who, like any independent unit of the system, will be required to respond to this essentially systemic event, regardless of her inner motivational stance. Matters of internal motivation and emotional readiness for a new type of relational contact may eventually move to the foreground, but not until there have been successful alterations of the structural positions of each family member.

With a structural diagnosis in hand, the therapist must then move to establish how all this relates to the family's request for help, what changes are envisioned, and who in the family needs to be involved in bringing them about. These are the topics of the next chapter.

Chapter 5

Opening Moves: Beginning New Structures

The initial interview does not end when the therapist arrives at a private structural diagnosis. That diagnosis must be translated back to the family members so that they may join the therapist in solving the problems that brought them to therapy. One step toward achieving this shared effort is for the therapist to redefine the meaning of the presenting problem—usually a symptom located in one person—by placing it in some larger set of events that involve the entire family system. It is initially a private move, made by the therapist, though later the family may be involved in some, and perhaps all, aspects of this redefinition. The point of changing the perspective on the problem, of moving from the single person to the family group, is to provide problem-solving leverage. It is not an effort to minimize the importance or meaning of the individual symptomatic behaviors.

THE SYMPTOM AND THE SYSTEM: MAKING THE SHIFT*

Structural family therapy assumes that there is a functional relationship between the troubled individual and the systemic operations of the whole family. Sometimes the relationship reflects incipient

*Parts of this chapter are based on Umbarger, C., & White, S. Redefining the problem: Individual symptom and family system. *International Journal of Family Counseling,* 1978, 6(2), 33–47, with permission.

disequilibrium in the family, as when Judy Fletcher tries to separate more from her mother. Then the symptomatic behavior serves to restore balance. At other times, the symptom points to a chronic homeostasis that consistently overwhelms any capacity for growth (as indicated in the summary comments on the function of Irving's symptoms in the Fletcher family). This assumption of a relationship between individual symptom and family system is a theoretical bias that must remain open to revision and refutation. For example, one can hardly suspect that every family with a troubled child is involved in some malevolent conspiracy to save the family by sacrificing the child. Indeed, most evidence points to a very different supposition: the current difficulties are often the ironic outcome of parenting strategies that were originally well intended. Structural family therapy distinguishes between the *origin* and the *maintenance* of a symptom. Moreover, some behaviors originate accidentally, as in cases of organic impairment or early histories of multiple foster-home placements. Whatever the circumstances and mystery of "origin," the structural family therapist observes the current family behaviors that reinforce and maintain the problem behavior. To redefine the problem can free the therapist from a search for original causes (and the concomitant, unhelpful hints of parental blame) and allow a focus on pattern-maintaining activities.

The idea of redefinition is sometimes confused with an actual dismissal of the presenting symptom. Haley (1977), in particular, has insisted that therapists focus almost exclusively on individual symptoms, leaving matters of redefinition entirely aside. This insistence reflected his increasing interest in the strategic, paradoxical, and hypnosis-related tactics that he believed could be applied to family problems. Structural therapy, in contrast, continues to be informed by a view of family functioning that includes the embeddedness of any single behavior in a larger chain of interactional events. Haley's concern that the therapist not overlook the original problem was, however, well founded, since redefining the presenting problem too often becomes only a variant of a more traditional warning that the patient's complaints are not the "real" problem. Actually, structural family therapy does take a position on the "real" problem; the family system is the locus of the real problem. This assignment is, happily, free of one burdensome connotation that usually accompanies any discussion of the "real" problem—the connotation of *depth* (that what is "real" is "deep" and things that are "deep" are more "real"). Historically, any warning that one is not dealing with the "real" problem carries with it the metapsychological assumptions of "depth" versus "surface." The warning suggests that painful presenting problems may only be a cover or, at best, a kind of surface condensation of the deeper, underlying problem. The implication of some psychoanalytic criticisms of family systems theory is that it addresses a superficial reality and that what is "deep" (i.e., inside an individual) is being overlooked in favor of the surface transactions of everyday life. If one can avoid these value-laden terms, then it is correct to say that when structural family therapists redefine the symptom in family terms, they move from the territory of intrapsychic imponderables (Rabkin, 1970) to the horizon of interpersonal transactions that occur in the relational (and hence, more observable) space of daily family life. (See Fig. 5-1.) From this viewpont, a symptom may have roots, if not origins, in aspects of the inner self as well as roots in the family system. Structural family therapy chooses to address the latter, assuming that when this is done, then inner-space correlates are also being altered, though in an indirect fashion.

Families are burdened with the same troublesome metaphysics, understandably preferring to locate the real problem as something residing entirely in one person and consigning that person to a space outside the boundaries of the family. The troubled person is frequently felt to be "out there" rather than "in here." A meaningful redefinition brings the problem back inside the living space of the family. It extends the boundaries of the family to include the symptomatic individual and rearranges the family's prevailing ideas of what is outside and what is inside. In this regard, the redefinition tampers with the family boundary between inside and outside, but it does so without introducing the complicating metaphor of depth, a word consistently associated with matters of individual psychology.

A redefinition of the symptom is only a restatement of the problem in terms of those recurrent family transactions that make possible continuation of the symptomatic behavior. It is never meant to be a dismissal of the subjective experience of families or of the concern for the symptomatic individual. It is meant to broaden the roster of *who* is included in the

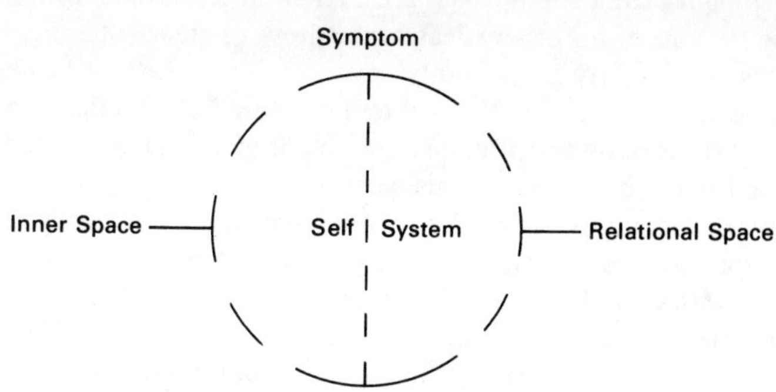

FIGURE 5-1. A diagram showing the relation of symptoms to self and system.

present-day affairs that are so disturbed. The goals of the redefinition are (1) to shift the focus from the individual to the family group; (2) to do this in such a way that the shift poses a solvable problem for both the therapist and the family; and (3) to make the new problem plausible and relatively benign rather than frightening and alienating. It is the therapist's task to define and demonstrate that a shift from individual symptom to family system is an efficient approach to solving the presenting problem.

WHAT TO TELL THE FAMILY

Whether or not to tell the family everything one thinks one knows about it is a surprisingly provocative issue. Those therapists schooled in theories of insight and/or humanistic enlightment seem to believe that to tell all is the best tactic for change and is, at any rate, ethically required. There are indeed serious ethical questions raised whenever a therapist chooses to withhold information from a family, especially since most people like to have some explanation as to why things have happened as they have, whether these explanations come from the therapist, from popular articles on psychology, or from other sources, such as religion. But there may also be ethical questions raised in an indiscriminate "telling all" to the family, since much of what a therapist thinks has only the status of unsupported hypotheses or, since we are all too human, the status of personal prejudice. More importantly, telling one's ideas to the family may actually be harmful when the therapist has been inducted into compliance with dysfunctional communicational structures. For example, telling a grandmother that she has too much power over her daughter and her grandchild may be a correct observation, but telling it *to* the grandmother inadvertently confirms this dysfunctional power hierarchy. In addition to these problems, some therapists share all their observations with the family because they have no other ideas about how to create change. In those instances, the tenacity of the family's problem is matched by the persistent, but futile chatter of the therapist, Jay Haley (1977) has admirably addressed some of these difficult issues, and interested readers may pursue the topic further by turning to his work.

For our purposes, we need only note that structural family therapists are cautious—especially in the beginning of therapy—not to overburden the client with complicated explanations, diagrams, or dramatizations of what the therapist believes to be the family's problem. While there is great respect for the client's "need to know" and a commitment to helping the family restructure its cognitive map of family life, structural therapists must always assume that the introduction of information into the family system is more than the simple communication of a content-message; the conveyance of information is simultaneously a metacommunication about the family's structural organization. This metacommunication may be an endorsement (either intentional or accidental), or it may be a challenge to the family's organizational structure. But it is never neutral and, consequently, can be harmful as well as helpful. Nowhere is this matter of "what to tell" more sticky than when the therapist attempts to usher into the family information that is intended to "redefine" for the family the meaning of its presenting problem. This, and other matters about what to tell the family, have been taken up by Minuchin and Fishman in their 1981 book. They have argued that a redefinition involves a direct challenge to the family's definition of the problem and a challenge to the family's notion of linear control. To make this challenge, Minuchin and Fishman have used highly cognitive approaches. They have suggested that the therapist become, in part, an expert witness. When the family says that Johnny, a soiler, is the problem, the therapist firmly replies that this is only partly true and that experience shows it requires total family participation to keep Johnny soiling. The therapist then directs the family members to begin talking among themselves about the problem and how they might contribute to it.

More important is the interruption of a family's assumption of linear control, that is, the notion that the family is being controlled by a single person, the index patient. "The therapist challenges the notion that one member can control the family system. Each person is rather the context of the other" (Minuchin & Fishman, 1981, p.196). In this spirit, Minuchin and Fishman have pushed for a redefinition based on the concept of reciprocity: that behavior is occurring in the context of back-and-forth exchanges with others. Such redefinition can be established, according to Minuchin and Fishman, by describing the behavior of one family member and then assigning the responsibility for that behavior to another family member. An example: "The therapist may say to an adolescent, 'You are acting like a four-year-old,' and then turn to the parents and ask, 'How do you manage to keep him that young?'" (p.197). Finally, again through quite educative steps, an attempt is made to challenge the family's epistemology "... by introducing the concept of expanded time, framing individual behavior as part of a larger whole" (p.197). Using this approach, the therapist will point out to the family that much of its behavior seems to obey rules that transcend any individual member. In this way, the therapist hopes to recast the symptomatic individual as simply one part of the larger family system, rather than an isolated individual who contains pathology.

The approach developed by Minuchin and Fishman involves giving the family most of the information about the therapist's cognitive schema.

Whatever one's personal stand might be on the "right to know" issue, there are some general guidelines that can be used when enlisting the family in a new view of the problem.

The principal tone to avoid in helping the family toward a different perspective is that which suggests that all family members are disturbed. When faced with such a "redefinition," they will either collectively confess that, indeed, as members of the human race, they too have problems (and thereby dismiss the therapist), or they will resist with even greater tenacity the plague being suggestively spread to them via the contaminating child whom they are already trying to isolate. The family either overaccepts or firmly dismisses redefinitions put in these general and clumsy terms. A successful redefinition, in contrast, is ushered in by: (1) presuming originally good intentions in all parties; (2) reframing the behaviors so that better personal identity imagery is available; (3) using the interview data to demonstrate that the symptomatic behavior can only occur in the context of other behaviors contributed by the family at large; and (4) using an "informational pathway" that is structurally correct for the family. Here are three examples of helpful and unhelpful efforts to redefine the meaning of the presenting problem.

The Jones Family: Louise and the Ghosts

Louise, age 16, was referred by her working-class parents because she was afraid of ghosts and, presumably in her desperation, hinted at suicide or mayhem as escapes from her terror. These hints were crayon drawings of daggers, dripping blood, and assorted gore, which Louise would leave outside her parents' bedroom door. She also was suddenly failing in school after years as an outstanding student. Her mother was herself a person of various transcendental experiences. She claimed to be clairvoyant and to be blessed with other extrasensory powers. The father was a mechanic, timid, clearly friendly toward Louise, and totally puzzled by the whole problem. There was one other child, a younger sister, age 11, who was without symptoms. During the interview, the mother revealed that she frequently spent the entire night sleeping in Louise's room to protect them both from harmful spirits. Louise would protest, saying she was too old for such nonsense, yet during the early evening, just before bedtime, she would begin her "artwork," as she tastefully called it. The mother would become alarmed, and the father would scold Louise, threatening to increase the already rather stringent limits on her social activities. During the interview, he tried to calm his wife's fears, agreeing with Louise that she was too old to believe in ghosts. His agreeing with Louise placed him in a coalition with his daughter against his wife, who, feeling herself possessed with special powers, resented his implicit skepticism. Consequently, the father typically fell silent in the interviews and at home typically went to bed shortly after the evening meal. Later, in the early hours of the morning, the father would awaken, hungry after his early retirement, and go downstairs to the kitchen where he made rather elaborate meals. He was generally joined in these early morning snacks by Louise, who herself seemed to awaken quite frequently, especially since she had become seized by her fears of ghosts. She and her father enjoyed a tasty and friendly time together before returning, some time before dawn, to their separate beds. The next day, Louise was frequently tired during the school day and, on several occasions, was sent home by the school nurse, who felt she looked pale and unwell. Near the end of the initial interview, the therapist offered to the family an elaborated view of the presenting symptoms. For comparison, two redefinitions are offered, one less suitable than the other, though both allude to nearly identical data.

FIRST REDEFINITION

Therapist: (Speaking to the mother) Your daughter leaves the drawings of blood and daggers and gore and so on, leaves them right by your bedroom door whenever you and your husband fight, and then you want to get comfort from her, like spending the night in her room. See, you are too dependent and don't want her to grow up. Because then, you would have to spend the night with your husband. So her drawings are a reminder that you need to first work things out in your marriage. That's the problem that first has to be solved.

SECOND REDEFINITION

Therapist: (Speaking to both parents) The two of you are correct in worrying about these drawings and in wishing that Louise would act more like her 16 years. I guess this happens when the two of you feel like she needs extra attention, such as when you, Mrs. Jones, spend the night in her room. What seems to happen is that *as parents* you get your signals mixed about how much support children need, and then, before you sort out your signals, one of you sort of moves ahead, like Louise was really in trouble. Then Louise has to find a way to push you back so she can be the more adult teenager you want. So she found out these drawings do that. And (speaking to Louise) you do a good job of reminding mom and dad that maybe they should ask you if you are feeling scared and needing help before they rush in.

Commentary

The first redefinition is unhelpful in several ways. It moves quickly to labeling the marriage as a troubled one, something that may be true but was not the reason for seeking help. It also labels the mother as "too dependent" and as a woman who does not want her daughter to grow up, again to protect her from the husband who, by implication, is represented as a disagreeable person. In their particulars, all of the assessments are probably correct: The marriage is troubled; the mother does want to avoid her husband; and she does depend on the daughter to provide her with a reason for avoiding him. But none of these points is phrased in such a way as to be acceptable to any family member. Moreover, the mother is singled out as the principal troublemaker.

In contrast, the second redefinition is directed to *both* parents, a move that avoids singling out the mother as though she were the guilty party. They are addressed in their *parenting* roles, not as marital partners. The therapist praises them for being concerned and suggests that they are in favor of Louise acting like a grownup. The problem is defined as one in which the parents get their "signals mixed," a polite way of pointing to some conflict about parenting. The problem description is continued by noting that one parent moves too quickly, a *timing error* rather than an issue of pathological intent. Louise's symptoms are depicted as a strategy she has developed in order to comply with the expectation which her parents, the therapist suggests, already have of her in the first place—namely, to act more independent of them, one sure sign of being more grown up. Finally, the therapist includes Louise in this expanded meaning of her symptoms by characterizing them as "reminders" to her parents that this is a matter of establishing better communication (they should ask first) and of better timing.

The Alfred Family: A Boy and His Mom*

Although only 18, Ken, the index patient, had been hospitalized repeatedly over the last four years. He was seen as highly disturbed, probably psychotic, with many assaultive tendencies. The usual object of his assaults was his stepfather, a man who had been with the family for 14 years. The family consisted of the mother, her three children by a first marriage, the stepfather, and an 11-year-old daughter by the current marriage. In addition to assaulting his stepfather, Ken became very regressed when he was around his mother, staying constantly by her side, touching her, showing anxiety and anger if her husband came near her. Ken and his mother exchanged many confidences, glances, and physical touches. They always sat together and indicated in many ways that theirs was the primary relationship in the family. There were many inappropriate

*This family is the subject of a training film, *Getting Out*, developed by Umbarger and Bernstein, The Family Institute of Cambridge (1979).

sexual overtones to their behavior. A family referral was made because, while Ken improved in the hospital, his behavior deteriorated rapidly after he returned home. The day before the family's initial interview, Ken and his older brother, Bill, had become involved in a physical fight with their stepfather, and Bill was thrown out of the house. The daughter fled to relatives, so only the parents and Ken showed up for the initial interview. After nearly 30 minutes of participation and observation, the therapist, a man, located a behavioral sequence he believed typical of this group. He intervened with a new definition of the problem, one involving all family members and not just the internal impulses of Ken. In a move to gather data, the therapist asked the two parents to talk together, something he observed had not yet happened in the interview. The parents began to argue about the children, with the stepfather raising his voice and the mother showing signs of fright. She spoke in a soft, tremulous manner, wrapping her coat tightly around herself. Their conversation continued in this way:

Stepfather: Everyone here says I'm beating up everybody.

Mother: And Kathy (a younger sister) is heartbroken because she loves you. . . .

Son: (Interrupting and turning to stepfather) We should. . . .

Stepfather: (Speaking angrily to Ken) Hey, look, would you let us talk? For Christ's sakes, you know. You know what you are? You just take from people and then you try to put me on the stand here, kiddo. You don't even know what's up and what's down.

Son: You're lying, and then you say . . . something like that. . . .

Stepfather: You know, you're in a world of fantasy.

Son: You're not, you're not. I don't like you (loudly, with rage).

Stepfather: I don't care if you don't like me. That doesn't bother me.

Son: (Leaning foward in a threatening way) I'll punch you in the mouth.

Stepfather: You won't ever touch me, fella. No. You and your brother won't touch me again 'cause I'll break your. . . .

Son: (Angrily interrupting) It comes to death now, motherfucker.

Stepfather: Don't call me your names, fella.

Son: I'll call Bill and have him knock you in the fucking head, or I'll do it myself. You fuck with him, I'll fuck with you.

Stepfather: (Threatening) Why don't you do that. . . .

The fight continued and became nearly out of hand. The therapist (moving later than he should have) finally asked them to stop and it took several minutes until the atmosphere cleared.

Therapist: Hey, stop. I want you to stop (said firmly, but without urgency). I want to teach you something. (The stepfather laughs.) Do you have any idea. . . .

Stepfather: (Interrupting) I'll laugh right in your kisser (said to the son).

Therapist: Do you have any idea how the two of you got into this fight?

Stepfather: He doesn't know what the hell is going on (said to the son).

Therapist: (Looking at the stepfather) Just hold on. (Then moving to the chair next to the son and addressing his comment to him) I'll give you an idea how you got into this fight . . . I'll tell you how you got into the fight . . . you do when your mother says she's helpless. When your mother indicates that she's trapped . . . , and she can't do anything. You get pulled into fighting at this time.

Son: Yeah?

Therapist: Yeah. And off you go.

Stepfather: Doctor, I don't fight with Ken.

Therapist: (To the stepfather) Oh, hold on a bit. (Turning to address the mother) But in a way, you know, you make this possible by throwing up your hands in helplessness. Now, you're grown up, and I would bet that you're able to deal with this guy (referring to her husband). You're a reasonable person. And that you can deal with this guy and that your son Ken does not have to come in and take over the action. That would be one observation. Hey, you see, I can see how, under other circumstances, the two of them would end up in a fist fight while you are acting more and more scared and quiet and helpless.

(Seconds later, the therapist adds to his comment) So the first order of business would be how you and your wife can fight in such a way that it doesn't involve these champions (alluding to his stepsons).

Stepfather: That's the way I feel.

Therapist: Like in olden times when knights used to be the champion of some lady.

Son: (Laughs in acknowledgement.)

Therapist: That's the way you and Bill are. You're your mother's champions in this jousting with the black knight.

Son: That's right. Yes.

Therapist: (Addressing the mother again) Lots of men fight over you. And you've got your sons and husband fighting over you. I can understand that, . . . and I also think that it's a serious concern and that you . . . one of the ways that you can stop this kind of jousting is by dealing more competently with your husband. (Moves his chair closer to the mother.)

Commentary

In this example, a critical interactional sequence is reported to the family as a redefinition of the presenting problem. The sequence involves the breakdown of contact between the parents when the mother signals she is frightened of her husband. She cues her son, who then interrupts the stepfather. A fight then develops between the son and stepfather, while the mother sits safely and silently by. While the stepfather wishes to label the son as crazy and living in a world of fantasy, the therapist attempts to teach the family a different viewpoint, one that shows how all three members contribute to this deadly sport of champions. The son seems relieved; the father agrees; meanwhile, the mother, typically, remains initially noncommittal, then suggests that she is too weak to fight with her husband. Her behavior is a matter for the therapy, not for the redefinition itself; that is, not all reframing moves must be wholly accepted by everyone in the family. Some resistance is naturally to be expected, in part because the first efforts at redefining will be only partially correct. At this point in the interview, the therapist at least has a purchase on a new definition of the reason for Ken's assaults upon his stepfather and has signs of some support from the family.

The Fletcher Family: The Men Who Help

Finding a workable redefinition was at first difficult for the Fletcher family's therapist. He did not want to share some of his hypotheses: that, for example, Mr. Fletcher was relatively powerless and peripheral, or that his wife had more emotional exchanges with her mother and her daughters than with him. These observations may have been correct, but each was in some way unpleasant and therefore would have been unwelcome to the family. Moreover, a good deal of what the therapist observed and inferred was no doubt already well known to the family. It was, for instance, probably no secret that Mr. and Mrs. Fletcher were relatively estranged from each other. To announce such would have been, at the very least, redundant and, more likely, would have been felt as an impolite infringement on the marital unit. After all, the Fletchers came for help with Irving, not with their marriage. But what else was true? What other broad perspective could the therapist have offered in order to diminish the scapegoating of Irving and achieve leverage for change throughout the total system? The therapist pursued the following alternative:

INTERVIEW	COMMENTARY
Therapist: Let me say what maybe is going on here. Because it's too late now and we should see about another meeting.	
1. (Speaking to both parents) You are right to be concerned about Irving, his	1. Concern for the presenting problem is validated.
2. trouble in school, and all. But (addressing the mother)	2. The therapist accommodates to the structural preference that new information be ushered into the family via the mother.
3. I think he has taught me	

4. something about your concerns for Judy. Because Irving, well, he doesn't want to take Judy's place with you. But he also knows how you worry about her being able to take care of herself. So his fighting with her sort of keeps her around, helping you out and everything until you are certain
5. she is ready to leave. And your husband is good about that too . . . staying out of your way until you can do the kind of job you did with the girls who are away. *He*
6. *understands a mother's job. So does Irving.*

3. The therapist makes an implicit alliance with Irving so that the mother is hearing Irving as well as the therapist.

4. A redefinition is tried. The mother's concern for her daughter becomes central. Irving's symptoms help the mother keep focused on Judy.

5. The husband is labeled as understanding, not peripheral.

6. Irving is labeled in the same way, implicitly joined to the father, a subunit that needs to be formed.

• • • •

Mother: I don't see . . . I . . . Judy is no worry to me. She's wonderful . . . no trouble. Only Irving.

Therapist: (Interrupting) But that's just it. You've done a good job with all your daughters, and she is wonderful. But partly you know that only because Irving gives Judy a chance to show how much she is *really* on your side.

The mother is both puzzled and resistant to the therapist's effort. She returns to worry about Irving. The therapist continues the effort, again suggesting that Irving's behavior is related to the mothering of Judy.

Judy: I am, mother. But I like it with Mary and Eileen, too. So that Irving just keeps dragging me back into the same old stuff.

This is an initial, though weak, indication that the reframing may hold some appeal.

Therapist: Tell your mother how that happens.

Judy: You get so upset. So I know . . . well, I'm the only one around. You can't talk to Mary or Eileen all the time. So it's me. That's O.K., but. . . .

The mother and daughter, in a critical dyad, are beginning carefully to air some of the tension in their relationship.

Mother:	But what? What are you saying?	
Judy:	I'm saying that I can't be around all the time, that you or Daddy or whoever got to make Irving stop. Because I can't worry all the time about your being upset.	
Therapist:	(To Judy) So you think your father should help your mother out with this . . . so that you. . . .	
Mother:	He doesn't know about this. He's not around at all. I can handle this.	The therapist has moved too quickly to bring the father into the parenting dyad. The mother is not ready to agree to his suggestion.
Therapist:	Then maybe you need to talk this over even more with Judy, to reassure her that you know how to handle this. Because she wants to grow up like her sisters.	Therapist retreats, going back to the unit already favored by the mother, but assigning a somewhat different task—namely, that the mother relieve Judy of her parental/child function and begin to plan ahead.
Mother:	Well, her sisters are older. They stayed right here until several years after school. Until their jobs were just right.	
Therapist:	So you already know that it will work out for Judy, then she can grow up like the sisters. And that you approve.	The therapist continues to press the theme of separation, but to normalize it, noting that the mother approves of growth.
Mother:	Yeah . . . I know it. I love her. I only want for her . . . to be ready.	
Therapist:	So now, you can tell Irving to let her alone, because you know how to get along without all your daughters at home. Tell him to stop doing you favors. Tell him to bother your husband instead. That you're doing O.K. with your end of the family.	In a critical move, the therapist again tries to enlist support for his view that Irving has been inadvertently helping the mother out. The mother is advised to treat this as a misunderstanding. Again, there is an effort to involve the father.
Father:	I can handle him. But I'm not around much.	The father's first entrance, mildly disqualified by himself.
Irving:	I don't need handling. I need to be left alone.	

Therapist:	Yeah, especially by your mother and sister. But that means you got to stop being so smart, I mean so sure that your mother doesn't know how to raise her daughters. She does, but she has her own time schedule.	The therapist supports the parental notion that Irving has to stop his bad behavior, but continues to label it as "smart," a phrasing that can be taken in two ways. He also suggests that the mother really does expect the daughters to grow away from her.
Irving:	Yeah, like forever.	
Father:	(To Irving) Don't get smart with your mother.	The father again enters, this time more firmly. It does not matter that he is opposed to Irving, only that he be dealing with him in some way.
Therapist:	(To the father) That's right; you handle that just for now. And, Mrs. Fletcher, I think I need another meeting with just you and these three older daughters. So you can discuss this time schedule about growing up.	The therapist sanctions the father-son dyad and proposes a treatment plan in accordance with this new view of the problem.

Commentary

This effort to free Irving from a scapegoated position seems moderately successful. The mother is not much impressed by the therapist's comments, and the father hardly rushes to take over. Still, Judy shows a stronger recognition of this formulation, and the father does participate a bit, imitating the therapist when he tells Irving not to get "smart with your mother." Above all, this effort demonstrates how a redefinition is, in fact, a restructuring intervention into the prevailing family operations. Regardless of the polite and supportive framing of each central point, the therapist is suggesting the presence of some future agendas that must be addressed (Judy's separation from her mother) and some new subunits that must be developed (father and sons). Resistance to this reformulation arises because everyone recognizes that some new arrangement of the family-force field is being proposed. The parents are also resistant because of the therapist's mistake in moving them together before they indicate any wish for that. Even greater resistance is avoided, however, because the therapist does not mention some of his initial assessments: that the mother, for example, is too enmeshed with her own mother; or that some of Irving's symptomatic behavior, especially at school with the male teachers, is an awkward strategy to bring his father more into contact with him and more inside the family. Although perhaps true, such notions touch the involved individuals too personally and too soon to be easily accepted. The mother would only defend her ties to her mother, and the father would doubtless insist that the therapist had failed to see that he really is running the family. Consequently, the redefinition process for the Fletcher family must move slowly, beginning with Irving's behavior as the gateway to commentary on the mother's dilemma about letting go of her adult daughters. When there is therapeutic progress in this area, additional aspects of the complete structural reframing may be successfully introduced.

TREATMENT GOALS, UNITS, AND STAGES

The initial phase of therapy draws quickly to a close when some reframing of the original problem has been achieved. The redefinition contains within it those goals of treatment that the family will endorse, the treatment unit most likely to solve the problem (not necessarily all the family members), and even some outline of the different stages in the treatment process. If the efforts at redefinition are successful, the therapist will have arrived at the treatment goals, units, and stages simultaneously.

Treatment Goals

The therapist and the family need to agree on why they would continue the meetings. Although they will not agree on all goals, they need to feel united on at least the major one. For example, in the case just cited of the boy who has assaulted his stepfather, the therapist, in his efforts to reframe the violence, comments, "So the first order of business would be how you and your wife can fight in such a way that it doesn't involve these champions." This is said to the stepfather and may be regarded as an initial goal of the subsequent therapy sessions. For the Fletchers, one of the initial goals is to convene the mother–daughter unit to achieve clarity about steps toward graduating from the family. A secondary goal—explicitly framed to add the mother, but implicitly intended to create another and new subsystem—is to join the father with the son so that the women in the family will not be distracted from their work by Irving's symptoms.

In general, the goals for treatment most likely to find support among family members are those that pertain to action, and specifically, action that bears on the presenting problem. Abstract goals—such as getting "better communication" or teaching people how to "express feeling"—are not likely to evoke more than conventional and polite support. We should all improve our communications and our emotional expressivity, no doubt. But in the crunch of meeting with a family, the initial interview phase should end with something that feels quite actively related to the stresses that prompted the visit.

The goals of treatment will change as the family moves through different stages of treatment. At the beginning, the goals will be behaviorally focused and will usually be about the index patient. Temporary coalitions and behavioral management problems may be suggested to provide the family with some respite from stress and to free them to focus on the related issues brought up during the process of reframing. In the Fletcher family, for example, the therapist suggests that the father act as the sole support and supervisor for Irving during the coming week—not because Mr. Fletcher is better suited for this role or because Mrs. Fletcher is incapable of it. The therapist makes this suggestion as a means of giving Mrs. Fletcher the freedom from worry that she needs in order to do a really good job of consulting with her daughters about Judy's separation from the family. In this way, small and immediate behavior goals are introduced so that other family members can pursue the expanded problem.

Treatment Units

Which members of the family will participate with the therapist in solving the problems they now agree are most pressing? Those implicated in the reframing process. As with the setting of goals, efforts to redefine and expand perspectives on the presenting problem automatically single out some family members as more crucial than others to the therapeutic process—at least at this stage. Of particular importance in this selection process is that no family member be totally excluded from some part in the healing process. Thus, while the therapist may require immediate meetings only with Mrs. Fletcher and her older daughters, he should emphatically mention to Mr. Fletcher and his son that their role is also important and that the therapist will look forward to the time he can meet with them and hear a report of their success in allowing the women to pursue their agendas.

It is most helpful during this beginning phase to have all family members present, including members of the extended family who seem to be involved. When all the players are gathered, the therapist and the family may generate scripts that do not require a full cast. Some family members can then be excused, at least for the first stage of treatment. It is much easier to see all possible participants at the beginning than subsequently to argue that other family members should be added for the next meeting. Parents are often reluctant to involve the "well" siblings or to let the extended family in on matters. Resistance is high, and the therapist has less leverage than is the case when the entire family has been gathered together at the beginning.

Finally, the conception of a treatment unit as composed of the therapist plus family members (Minuchin, 1974) must be maintained. The active presence of a therapist forces the family to create a new system, one that by design and therapeutic intent upsets the customary equilibrium and requires the family to form a new unit with at least some new rules. In a sense, the most fundamental requirement for change is that the new unit break some rules of the old one. When the therapist joins in such a way that therapeutic rule breaking occurs, there is a chance for change. When the joining process breaks no rules, there is only induction into the preexisting family system.

Treatment Stages

The treatment process benefits when the therapist can envision an evolution of stages, a progression from one treatment unit solving its special problem to a subsequent unit with its special issues, and, in some instances, to the reconvening of the entire family at various points in the treatment. As already noted, not all problems will require the presence of the entire family at each therapy session; instead, different problems may require the convening of different subgroups within the family. When therapists can plan the probable order in which to meet with these subunits, they have at the same time planned the treatment stages.

The chief advantage of this staging is to make acceptable the transitional imperfections in working arrangements with the family. For example, suppose the initial problem is the dilemma of an overfunctioning mother and an underfunctioning father, the object of these efforts being the child whose symptoms provide the occasion for each parent to play his or her role. In the initial stage of treatment, the therapist might arrange for the parents to keep their role behavior in full swing, but might redirect it toward some adult members of their extended family (e.g., the wife's mother). A critical observer would be quick to point out that the mother-in-law would now become enmeshed in her daughter's overfunctioning behavior. The alternative view, however, would be that the transitional treatment stage is less harmful than the original family oganization that focused on the child. The child is less able to cope with the parental conflict than an adult, the mother-in-law, who will be more able to withstand the enmeshments of her daughter and the ineptitude of her son-in-law. Most certainly, the therapist must next move them all to another stage of treatment that more directly confronts this particular marital dynamic.

This example shows that transitional stages of therapy are imperfect, but they are less imperfect than the chronic family organization originally encountered by the therapist. Each succeeding stage should allow the family to move toward a healthy structure that is congruent with the family's value preferences and membership in the surrounding community.

Staging therapeutic interventions also reduces resistance and is respectful of a simple, but powerful reality: the family is generally stronger than the therapist, and its system will not gently or easily be rearranged by an outsider. This is not because families mean to resist, but because it is the nature of systems to resist *radical* change. Intervening is like a game of Pick-Up-Sticks: one must be thoughtful about the structure one touches lest all around it be pushed to a state of imbalance too great to sustain the game. Some breathlessness is part of the process, but as in the game of Sticks, the therapist must tease the whole apart while maintaining constant respect and regard for the adjacent pieces. No part of a system can be precipitously moved without reverberations throughout the member parts. One must therefore *stage* the therapeutic rearrangement in a manner designed to move the family to new levels of structural operation, not to renewed resistance or rigidification of function.

Using the Fletchers as an example, Table 5-1 shows some possible treatment stages suggested by the initial management of the presenting

Table 5-1
HYPOTHETICAL PLAN SHOWING POSSIBLE TREATMENT STAGES IN THE FLETCHER FAMILY

Stage	People Involved	Problem and Goal
1	Mother and daughters	Judy, in her response to Irving, is overinvolved with the mother in a coparenting dyad. This slows her movement to the outside world, as represented by the older sisters. This stage of therapy will reassure them all that the mother can promote Judy's exit as she did for the others.
2	Father and sons	The Fletcher men are only loosely federated. The goal of this stage is to solidify their identity as men and as a subgroup within the family.
3	Sibling group	There is some estrangement between the brothers and sisters. If they could develop themselves as a cohesive group, it would force the parents into a separate unit.
4	The "at-home" family: parents, Judy, Irving, and Janice	The parenting unit needs to be redefined as one excluding Judy. The problems of Irving and Judy must be dealt with by the mother and father together, with some emphasis on the father's greater presence.

problem. It would be ideal if stages 1 and 2, as outlined in Table 5-1, could occur simultaneously. The men could be forming their subunit while the Fletcher women are articulating theirs into those who are to remain appropriately at home—the mother and the youngest daughter, Janice—and into those mature enough to be primarily identified with the extrafamilial world. The focus of the sibling group recognizes that both Irving and Judy are overinvolved with the mother and underinvolved in the other units that would give them a different sense of personal direction and identity; Irving needs to be more with his brother, Bob, and less at war with his sisters. They all need to experience something in common *as siblings distinct from their parents.* This experience affirms a group identity appropriate to the family's life cycle issues and, as an indirect spinoff, forces the mother and father into a clearly defined space as occupants of the parental subunit. The exclusion of a treatment stage involving only Mr. and Mrs. Fletcher presumes that they do not themselves raise obvious marital issues and that their difficulties in coparenting are addressed in the above format. It is equally likely that one may see them alone in their role as *parents*, without the children. That would be useful and, in that context, they may raise some questions about their married life. Finally, convening the whole family provides a chance to help the now more articulated subunits transact business with each other, including differences of opinion. If possible, a focus on the parenting of Janice, age 10, will position the parents to do more with each other while freeing the older children to continue their progress toward the outside world.

The issues of treatment units and stages have been briefly presented here; they obviously represent a major intervention strategy into family functioning through the intentional rearranging of subgroups. How the therapy is conducted during these stages of treatment is the concern of the next two chapters. Those chapters explore what therapists should do once they have arranged a treatment goal and a family group willing to meet with them at this particular stage of the process.

Chapter 6

Classic Interventions: Structure, Staging, and Sequence

By the end of the initial interview, there has been a good deal of active contact with the family. They have been convened as a whole, yet also divided into subgroups as part of the structural assessment. Their initial concerns have been granted credibility through placement in a larger family process, an event called *redefinition*. Treatment goals have been agreed upon, and a group of family members has been selected to work on these goals. It remains to be seen whether or not this initial burst of activity is any more than the therapeutic equivalent of reshuffling deck chairs aboard the Titanic. When the activity clearly facilitates the process of structural family therapy, some ordered change may now unfold. Beyond the initial interview lies the dogged, usually undramatic, process of bringing about the changes that seem needed. This chapter and the ones that follow describe some of the standard moves made to bring about change. Some thoughts about family resistance to change are also discussed; as is the issue of what to do after good moves fail.

Altering family structure to produce some temporary flux or crisis in the system is a necessary first step in the process of change. As noted in Chapter 2, a system close to its maximum point of equilibrium is less ready for alteration than one operating far from equilibrium. Hoffman (1981), Caille (1979), Dell (1982), and Glansdorff and Prigogine (1971) have all observed that the homeostatic rigidity of pathological systems must be disrupted before more adaptive structural transformations may occur. In a sense, all of the intervention strategies reviewed below, as well as being instrumental in the reinforcement of new structures, may be used to create just such a system crisis. Minuchin has described various such strategies,

(Minuchin & Fishman, 1981) and they are recast and summarized here as the "classic" interventions of structural family therapy. When structural therapists who are beginning this work have mastered these classic moves, they will no doubt wish to reach for the kinds of refinements described by Minuchin in his more recent work (Minuchin & Fishman, 1981). The intention here is to familiarize the reader with the broad categories of interventions used throughout the course of structural therapy. Because these moves are perhaps first apparent in efforts to unbalance the family's pathological system, thereby inducing some level of crisis, the place of crisis in relation to change needs some brief elaboration.

PROVOKING A CRISIS

A therapist, as noted earlier, may be characterized as an *active joiner*, a *systems irritant*, and a *therapeutic rule breaker*. These labels are reminders that the therapist joins the family group in such a way that a new system is formed—the *therapeutic system*. It consists of the family plus the therapist. The immediate goals of this new system are to introduce novelty, variety, and diversity into the family's strategies for living and to substitute them for the programs of constancy, control, and chronic routine that characterize the pathological system. This push for flux and novelty in the family's routines is consistent with a general systems view that increased diversity and complexity signals a healthy organization. The therapist, as the active agent for change, has a responsibility to induce the critical instabilities that will allow such complexity to emerge.

Minuchin has provided a helpful distinction between crisis and emergency (Minuchin & Barcai, 1969). The latter refers to the routine and fruitless problem-solving efforts applied to chronic states of stress. A genuine crisis, on the contrary, occurs when these usual strategies for stress reduction have been challenged and blocked. A crisis is really the unsettling stress of being required to solve problems in a new way. A family crisis sometimes occurs naturally as, for example, in times of sudden unemployment or in the unexpected death of a family member. But the more common situation confronting a therapist is one in which the family compounds its many serious problems with coping strategies that are even more crippling than the original presenting symptoms. In these instances, where there is no natural crisis, the active therapist may create a crisis for the family by (1) persistently interrupting some critical behavioral sequences until new problem-solving routines emerge; (2) by restructuring certain family subsystems, thereby breaking some critical family rule that maintains the problem (for example, restructuring the Fletcher family groups so that the father and his sons form a stronger subgroup); and (3) by a deliberate staging of family-group behavior such that those members involved in handling an emergency are replaced by other members who are ordinarily peripheral to the problem. For instance, an overinvolved mother may be deflected from attending to the emergency of a daughter with cyclical vomiting when the therapist instead requires that the daughter be assisted by an older sib in cleaning up the vomit, replacing fluids, and so forth. The mother, during these times, is asked to phone her husband (the parent usually not involved) at work and discuss with him her many anxieties and concerns that, without her, the symptomatic daughter's illness will become worse. Such a restaging of the family's usual response to chronic emergency is an intermediate step in the therapy, a step designed to create new stresses in the parenting unit and hence new opportunities for change.

When a crisis occurs, even a brief one, the therapist must often be on call for the puzzled and sometimes frightened reactions of the family. In a period of flux, there is a brief loss of old stabilities. No new assurances are in sight. Everyone is upset, and no one can imagine how the situation will improve. When crisis induction is undertaken, therapists must be ready to handle late evening and weekend phone calls, to arrange for extra therapy sessions when needed, and most importantly, to have the support of their colleagues. Crisis induction is not easily accomplished. When it succeeds, the therapist must then offer considerable support and facilitation for the new problem-solving behaviors that develop. The techniques for crisis induction may be drawn from any of the classic interventions described below and in the next chapter. To these matters we now turn.

SEEING THE STRUCTURE

Structural family therapy is a state of mind as well as a compendium of techniques. Precedence is generally given to the pursuit of structure rather than to psychological content, except when a discussion of the psychological meaning of a behavior is used as an intentional strategy for joining. Some systems will not admit a therapist unless some sympathetic review is given to the psychological sophistication of those family members who have previously been in therapy or been analyzed. This review of psychological content, however, is not so much pointless as premature. When the structuring of a family's strategy for information exchange is not addressed, the informational content remains bound in dysfunctional behavioral sequences and is not, in itself, sufficient to bring about change. Thus, the structural therapist attempts to target all interventions toward the structuring strategies characteristic of the family, not toward the psychological content that the family offers. The case of Mrs. N's genogram, as described in Chapter 1, is an illustration of this emphasis.

The reader may recall that one problem the therapist needed to address was how the seven-year-old daughter would interrupt and cling to her mother whenever the mother began to talk about her own problems. There were two kinds of remarks the therapist could make at that point: one distinctly structural, and an alternative comment that was primarily psychodynamic (see Table 1-1, p. 5). As noted in Chapter 1, however correct in purely psychological terms the alternative remark might be, it does nothing to alter the interactional sequences that bind together mother and daughter. From a structural viewpoint, the two remarks have the impact shown in the symbolic diagram on page 5. In this example, the pursuit of psychological content, which might be helpful at another time, now only continues the original pathogenic family organization. This argues for the usefulness of seeing structural issues first, altering them, and then where necessary, pursuing matters of more traditional psychodynamic interest.

STAGING AS AN INTERVENTION

Staging has two general meanings. First, it is the deliberate arrangement of a natural system into either its existing components or into new groupings so that the therapist achieves leverage for change. In this way, staging may be accommodating (focusing on the subdivisions that already exist) or restructuring (creating new and unfamiliar subdivisions in the family). Second, to stage either an interview or an entire treatment procedure means an active planning of what to do first, second, third, and so on. To talk about a stage of treatment simply designates a particular set of therapeutic operations as time-limited and acknowledges that a different set of therapeutic efforts will eventually replace the current ones. For example, one often stages the introduction of some specific behavioral change, as when parents may be counseled to let their son continue his temper tantrums, but to require him now to extend the amount of time that these tantrums usually take. At a later stage, they may be asked not only to let him keep some records of the time spent in tantrum behavior, but to require as well that he now announce when he is going to have one. This is the staged implementation of a single intervention.

The case of the Fletcher family highlights the other kind of staging: the selection of different family subgroups to focus on different aspects of the total system problem. The Fletcher case, in fact, went through a number of stages. Not all cases treated by a structural approach do so. Indeed, many cases, such as those involving a small number of family members or those with certain types of presenting problems, may never break into subgroups, but may meet as a total unit for every session. The provision of a separate meeting time for one part of the family can, however, be a powerful message about the restructuring needed. Simply meeting with Mr. Fletcher and his two sons, for example, would convey to the family that it needs to reorganize itself so that the men can experience more alliances with each other. Another common move is to meet with the couple alone, thereby supporting their right to a marital life separate from their parental duties. Staging can ensure that the therapeutic context will embody—in its formal structure—the content of structure actually discussed by family and therapist.

While staging can be carried out with these large strokes, it can be used with equal effectiveness within a single interview. This staging within one interview mirrors the larger movements, but makes for more immediate impact. Any division of the single meeting into segments in which some family members are central and others are peripheral may be considered a staging intervention. Consider the following case examples.

The parents of an unmanageable four-year-old girl complained that the mother could handle her only when her husband was present to support her. In block play, this seemed verified when it came time to clean up the blocks: the mother struggled with her daughter, but only with the husband's encouragement did she get the daughter to comply. Since the husband could not be home all day, the mother had to learn to manage by herself, setting aside for the moment whatever message about the marriage she might covertly have been sending to her husband. Therefore, the therapist asked the husband to wait outside while the mother and daughter started a new game. During this stage of the interview, the therapist was completely passive in order to avoid simply taking the husband's role. The therapist observed how the mother let herself be defeated by a small child. In a third stage of this single interview, the therapist might have considered sending the child out to her father and then passing on to the mother the observations that were made and the suggestions for change that these observations implied. Finally, if time allowed (or for the next session), the mother and daughter might take up a game, this time with the mother practicing the new tactics discussed with the therapist. In a 60-minute interview, then, it would be possible to go through all four stages: (1) parents plus child; (2) mother and child alone; (3) mother with therapist; and (4) mother and child again alone, using the therapist's input.

In another case, that of the Darcy family, both parents and the oldest son were alcoholic, and the mother was very enmeshed with the youngest son, a 21-year-old schizophrenic named Sid. In the beginning of the second interview, a staging maneuver occurred when the therapist attempted to separate the mother from the son and let his father move in. This dialogue is testimony to the rigidity of the family pattern:

Therapist: Mrs. Darcy, I would like for you to sit over here next to me, relax for a while, and let Sid talk to his father.

Mother: No, . . . he's afraid of his father. They. . . .

Son: I never talk to him, no, I never. . . . No, I never. . . .

Father: Oh, I always let his mother handle him. She. . . .

Mother: I understand Sid better, so we agree that. . . .

Therapist: (Interrupting everyone) You're all so cozy about this, that Sid and his father never talk. It's like a rule you have: Sid is to be afraid of his father. I want to break that rule. Go ahead, Mr. Darcy. Ask Sid about coming to the hospital's day program.

Son: (To the therapist) I think I'm getting sick, my stomach hurts. I need something to eat. Are my ears funny to you? Are you laughing at me?

Therapist: Your ears are for listening to your father. That's the only task now, for the two of you to talk together. For five minutes only. Your mother is prohibited from talking, so you are on your own. (To the mother) If you interfere, I will ask you to leave the room for five minutes. If you can't let them have five minutes without you, especially with me right here, then your family is really stuck.

Son: I don't know what to say to him.

Therapist: That's all right, 'cause during this stage of things, your father is going to take the lead. Go on, Mr. Darcy. Help your son get going.

Father: Oh, he's my baby. He knows I won't hurt him. Right, Siddy dear? (Blows a kiss to his son.)

Therapist: Now you are acting like your wife, you are keeping her right here so she is still having to work with her son. Don't baby him like your wife does. He's not a baby. (To Sid) They make you a baby, and you make them successful at it by acting dopey. (To the father) Try it again. We still have a few minutes left before your wife comes back to take over.

At this point, the father and son succeeded in exchanging relatively empty reassurances about the hospital day program. They did so looking directly at each other and without reference to Mrs. Darcy, who continued to remain silent, sitting next to the therapist.

In this example, the establishment of a stage that excluded the mother required considerable effort. It finally succeeded for only a few minutes. (This same example also illustrates task setting in a single interview, where the task is to endure a restructured alliance system for a five-minute period.) The therapist had to persist and use forceful language to pry the family into a new arrangement. Actually, a second stage was automatically set up, for at the end of the five-minute period, the mother would be allowed to rejoin the group, free of any instructions or restraints. The therapist would then observe closely how she reentered and note if the family group carried on in exactly the manner it did before the stage that excluded her.

CHANGING THE HIERARCHY

When therapists stage interventions, they often do so as a means of addressing gross problems in the family's hierarchical arrangements. As each stage of an intervention is successfully completed, there is the corresponding hope that problems in the distribution of power and influence will also be gradually corrected. A dominant reality of all organizations is that some hierarchical arrangement of the component parts—some design for different levels of functioning, such that some levels are higher up and more influential than other levels—is invariably necessary if the organization is to thrive. Haley (1980) has presented some excellent thoughts on this matter and has based his most recent work on the necessity of reordering confused hierarchies.

To challenge a confused power hierarchy, Minuchin and Fishman have used a technique called "unbalancing" (1981, pp.161–190). Also called intentional "therapeutic side taking," this technique seems useful for cat-like systems that resist any type of therapeutic intrusion and regain balance regardless of any momentary flux in their pattern. Minuchin and Fishman have pointed out that in one way the hierarchy of the family is already broached when the therapist is admitted as an expert and therefore *above* the others. Families will generally tolerate this inequality as long as their own hierarchy is not challenged. Using a capacity for affiliation, the therapist can offer an unequivocal alliance with a family member or a subsystem and persist in that alliance until the system is pushed into crisis and change. Such side taking is a delicate business. It works when it works, that is, whenever the family member or subsystem accepts this strong alliance and allows it to open new possibilities. This is not a tactic long endured by anyone, including the family member who receives this special affiliation and who enjoys the benefits only while risking the disfavor of others. According to Minuchin and Fishman, the therapist ". . . must continue stressing the system in order to produce a transformation, but he must also be aware of feedback indicating whether the family members are able to follow him in the exploration of new alternatives in their transactions" (1981, p.187). When new sequences are started, the therapist needs to repair some fences and restore affiliations with other family members.

In the following example, unbalancing was used after several months of failure with other interventions. The family's hierarchy was confused in two ways. First, the husband, through unemployment and eccentricity, had joined the subgroup of his two sons, who themselves were identified primarily through odd behaviors. This left the mother a virtual single parent. Secondly, however, the family was not run by this "single parent," but instead was dominated by the subgroup that consisted of the two symptomatic children and the father. It seemed necessary to get the father firmly relocated in the parenting system in which he would cooperate with his wife in managing the two children. After several months of failure to achieve this hierarchical regrouping, the therapist tried unbalancing the stuck, dysfunctional hierarchy. Here is how it worked.

The Link Family: Dracula in Orbit

Mr. Link was a tall, sparse man of almost 40 years of age. He had been unemployed for several years, having left a promising job as a professor of geology in order to shift his attention from the planes of the earth to those of the heavens. He now devoted all his time to designing a game of "Orbits" in which the players attempted to plan orbital trajectories of planets around a mythical sun such that each planet would be warmed into life, yet not collide with each other or be fatally drawn into the sun. The family was supported by Mrs. Link, a timid and sensible woman who worked part-time as an assistant printer. The oldest son, age 18, had been diagnosed as a paranoid schizophrenic. He spent considerable time dressed as Dracula and staying in his room, which he referred to as his "earthen crypt." When he emerged, it was to help his father plan the game of "Orbits." The youngest son, age 11, was diagnosed as a behavior problem and was in a special school. In working with the couple so that they might be better positioned to help their sons, the therapist found them hopelessly deadlocked. They described their relationship as "like tepee poles," each person able to be partially erect only because he or she leaned on the other for support. As such, when Mrs. Link suggested a number of good ideas about the management of her sons, she was always undercut, gently, by her husband, who would threaten to collapse his side of the tent. Mrs. Link would then back down and comply with her husband's preference for stability. Stasis reigned supreme.

After some weeks of this deadlock, the therapist, a man, entered into unequivocal support of the wife, siding with her on all issues and finally encouraging her to make more of a separate career for herself in interior design, an aspiration she had long nurtured. During the sessions, the therapist would enter into long discussions with Mrs. Link about her ideas and aspirations and make concrete suggestions about additional training. Only at the end of the interview, while ushering the couple out, would he speak to the husband, generally to bid him goodbye and thank him for letting his wife move ahead.

After the third such meeting, the couple arrived with Mr. Link in a fury at the therapist. He was angry that the therapist had displaced him. He felt accused of being unable to promote his wife's interests. As evidence to the contrary, he had spent the last week redesigning a part of their house to be a studio for her. He had abandoned his own game-planning activities in order to have enough time to build new shelves for her pens and inks and to put a skylight in the studio. His wife was very appreciative, but persisted in her career goals rather than be swept back into compliance with his readiness to continue their marginal life. A true fight began between the couple, with the husband now fully committing himself to share his fears and disappointments about their family life. The therapist was able to monitor this as an impartial observer, friendly to both sides. As the husband became joined with his wife in this new way, they then, as a unit, regained an executive position in the family hierarchy. This change represented a new, healthier balance in the hierarchy between children and parents and was the response to the state of unbalance created by the therapist when he placed the considerable weight of his position entirely on the wife's side.

SEEING A SEQUENCE

Hierarchies exist and are maintained by the repetition of discrete behavioral cycles called sequences. A *sequence* has no particular status as a psychological construct; it is simply a word used to designate a collection of interpersonal behaviors that, taken as a cybernetic whole, constitute a dynamic entity that regularly appears in the family's life process. Another practical synonym for *sequence* might be *strategy,* a word indicating that these behaviors are organically coherent and achieve some larger goal in the family system. For example, a sequence of behaviors noted for the Fletcher family involved the index patient and his older sister in a type of fight that helped the mother to stay firmly allied with her daughters and estranged from her husband. The larger systems goal—the maintenance of strict subunit boundaries between men and women—was well served by these repetitive fights. The fight activity was the strategy used by the Fletchers to achieve that goal. Such sequences or strategies are the dynamic stuff of hierarchical structures and subunit boundaries. Consequently, many clinicians feel the most important business of therapy is to alter those sequences. Haley comments, for example, that the ". . . goal of therapy is to change the sequences that occur among people in an organized group" (1977, p.105).

Before one can interrupt sequences, several difficult questions need attention. What is the relationship between sequence and structure? How does one see a sequence? What is the place of sequences in a systems view of family process? Although these are obviously quite complex questions, some brief answers will at least help the clinician begin to relate sequence to therapeutic change. First, a note on the relation of sequence to structure. (The reader is also referred to the earlier discussion of structure and content in Chapter 1.)

Relating Sequence to Structure

Structure is the summary of a sequence. Which structure emerges, in our mind's eye and in diagram, depends on where one punctuates the sequence. Structure is sequential process made static. Like a child's game of Statues, a structure is the tableau obtained when one freezes the whirl

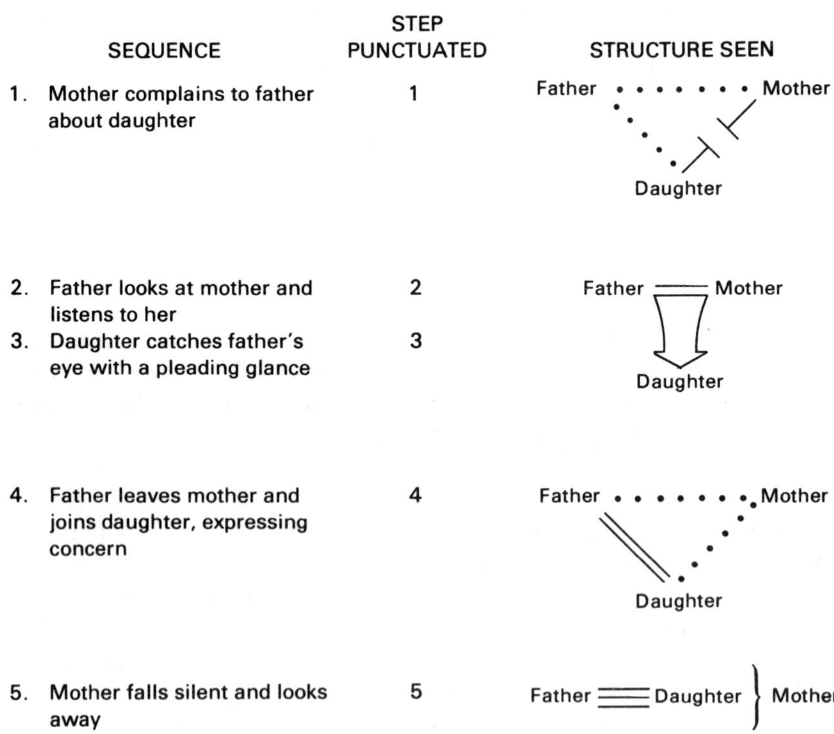

FIGURE 6-1. Possible relationships between sequence and structure.

of process. Stopped here, one sees a "statue" misaligned, arms akimbo, balancing on a single leg, an expression of perhaps both amusement and anger on the player's face. Stopped there, at another point in time, the "statue" is firmly balanced on both feet, arms extended in comfortable welcome or crossed in the firm integrity of splendid isolation. In the game, "statues" appear when one shouts, "Stop," and the players oblige. In therapy, structure appears when the therapist punctuates a sequence, deciding silently that a "stop" has occurred. Just as when to shout, "Stop," is the crux of an amusing game of Statues, so too is the timing of sequence punctuation a crucial determinate of the structure one sees.

Envision the possible interchanges between sequence and structure occurring in the abstract example shown in Figure 6-1. The difference in "seen structure" between punctuating at step 1 and step 5 is considerable. In step 1, only the antagonism between the mother and daughter is evident, other relationships remaining obscure. At step 5, there are cumulative, and thus convincing, indications of a more frequent and enduring structure: the father and daughter are in an enmeshed dyad that forms a coalition against the mother, who now appears extruded and peripheral. Since different structures may be seen at different points of sequence punctuation, the therapist may well feel confusion, if not despair, as to *when* in interactional time one assumes the punctuation of process. Despite the apparent opportunities for multiple punctuations, one's task is actually easier than it might first appear. Consider these two points:

1. Interactional process in families varies in rhythm, tone, or temper. Family process has rhythms, tonal variations, and cosmetic changes, like an organism that breathes in and out, punctuating the end of an exhalation with a small pause before beginning to inhale. Since process is marked with such pauses, it is useful to imagine that process consists of linked loops of interactional behavior.
2. These loops are what one means by *sequence*. There are only a few steps in each sequence loop. Not dozens, but a few.

In summary, the interactional process is like a series of interconnected bridges that carry the family from event to event, filling experiential time with the family walkways of behavioral routines. These bridges are the sequences that interest us. Each such bridging sequence consists of only a few parts or steps. When one bridging sequence is ended and another ready to enter, the therapist will experience a suspension of movement, in the family as well as in oneself. This pause signals the best place to punctuate a sequence, extracting from that punctuation a structure that will serve as a guide to intervention strategies.

Obviously, nature does not arrange itself in quite such an orderly fashion, and the whole business of when something starts and ends may be most complicated. Bridges are nice in their concreteness, but as metaphors they may oversimplify a very complex event. Still, the therapist is helped by such metaphors and by a common observation—namely, that some "things" (sequences) seem to keep happening over and over. This repetition, and the therapist's experience of it, are two events which make it possible even to dare to represent life's complexities in terms of metaphors and assumptions that something has "stopped" (been punctuated). Nature's process may not be tidy, but thankfully it is filled with redundancies. These redundancies are the critical sequences in family process. One learns to see them, to recognize the essential steps in them, and to know when "Stop" has been shouted, thus punctuating and transforming the sequence into a structural picture that will itself suggest some therapeutic intervention.

Finding Sequences

When one has considered the relationship of sequence to structure and the role of sequences in family process, the question still remains, "How does one find them?" In becoming ready to "see" sequence, the therapist needs that special stance discussed in Chapter 3, the stance of the pinball player. This stance allows one frequently to retire from active participation in order to observe the ritual exchanges among family members. To see sequence, the therapist needs to assume this role of observer as well as, later on, the role of director of the family's drama. The honing of this observational skill is essential in seeing and sensing routine sequences of family behavior. The frequent viewing of videotapes of family interviews is often helpful in acquiring this skill.

There are, in addition to this general stance, some specific tips that indicate when one is face-to-face with a sequence. These include the following:

1. When a sequence is finished, punctuated by the family itself (before taking another interactional breath), the therapist can experience this pause as a moment of transactional blankness, a time when it seems that things have ended and nothing else has begun. The family may be quiet, frozen, emotionally struck, or even obviously finished, perhaps labeling the significant end of the sequence by complaining, "See, this is always how it turns out!"
2. The therapist recognizes the outcome of some behavioral exchange before it actually arrives. The story has been told before.

3. An interesting comment made by the therapist has been digested by the family in such a way that even the therapist forgets the remark.
4. A variation of the "lost remark": when a sequence has not yet run through its cycle, efforts by the therapist to intervene will fail. The family will override the intrusion (unless it is very strong), thereby alerting the therapist that a sequence is in progress.
5. Asking the family to describe how things unfold can give valuable clues to the steps in a sequence by noting who says what to whom, who responds next, what happens then, etc. This is a kind of tracking of the family's report of the behaviors that seem to lead to some particular stopping place in the family's life.

Finding Macrosequences

In addition to being a good observer and mastering such tip-offs, the therapist must be ready to develop a scenario of sequences that fits the events as adequately as possible and should not wait for some sign to confirm that the details of the scenario are absolutely correct. These scenarios may be written large or small. Haley (1977) has given excellent examples of scenarios describing family events that occurred across rather large periods of time—hours or even days. His analyses of macroscopic sequences also involved attributions of competent and incompetent behavior. Here is one example involving two generations:

1. One parent, usually the mother, is in an intense relationship with the child. The mother attempts to deal with the child with a mixture of affection and exasperation.
2. The child's symptomatic behavior becomes even more extreme.
3. The mother or the child calls on the father for assistance in resolving their difficulty.
4. The father steps in to take charge and deal with the child.
5. The mother reacts against the father, insisting that he is not dealing with the situation properly. The mother may react with an attack or a threat to break off the relationship with the father.
6. The father withdraws, giving up the attempt to disengage the mother and the child.
7. The mother and the child deal with each other in a mixture of affection and exasperation until they reach a point where they are at an impasse.

And the sequence begins again. Haley has noted that disturbances in hierarchies come about through repeated sequences of behavior that involve coalitions of members from different levels of the hierarchy who, from that vantage point, perform activities against a third person. The behaviors in any particular sequence, he has suggested, always reflect a hierarchical problem if cross-level coalitions are present, as in the example above. In Haley's sequence examples, there is a minimum of three steps and usually more, and at least two generations of family members are required. Haley has advised that the disturbed hierarchy, and the sequences which support it, can be changed when the therapist prevents coalitions across generation lines.

In addition to such advice about specific goals for each interview session, locating these macrosequences can assist one in long-range treatment planning. If, for example, the index patient routinely provokes a hospitalization whenever the parents discuss a summer vacation, then the therapist is alerted to the probability of such a sequence repeating itself as the summer approaches. It is often easier for the beginning therapist to locate these broad programs of family life rather than to see the sequences that are the stuff of moment-to-moment exchanges among family members.

Finding Microsequences

More difficult to observe are the microscopic transformations of these larger behavioral plans, the brief and rapid series of events that occur right before one's eyes in the heat of the interview. Often these brief flurries are *isomorphic transformations* of larger sequences; both have the same form, follow the same rules of order, and hence are structural equivalents of each other. If one can spot and decipher the rules of a large sequence, it is likely that some transformation of it will be played out during momentary exchanges within the actual interview. *Induction* is the therapist's unwitting participation in these isomorphs. He ignorantly plays one of the part-steps in the total sequence and thereby finds himself involved in furthering some dysfunctional process. Consider this example. During one stage of an interview, a father talked with his mildly retarded, semidelinquent adolescent son about how the son would get to his daily treatment program.

Father: So do you know how to use the bus, to get from home to here (indicating the hospital)?

Son: I know that buses come here.

Father: Yeah, but . . . look at you, at your trip here. Do you know which bus to catch? And will you really do it? (Some irritation is apparent in father's voice.)

Son: I know some kids whose parents drive them all over. And then there's a long walk from some bus stops to here.

Father: Now you are simply not listening. How can I feel sure you can take the bus when you won't even talk about it here. (The father looks at the therapist.) See! This is the way he gets at home . . . just vague, so we don't know . . . (sounds angry).

Son: (He puts on a pair of dark sunglasses and looks out the window. He remains silent.)

Therapist: I think your father really wants you to succeed at this bus thing. Ted, can you look at your father? (The son continues to look out the window and remain silent.)

During this natural pause, this clear punctuation of their efforts at discussion, the therapist formulated a four-step sequence that had, one could see in retrospect, appeared at other points in the father's effort to talk with his son. The sequence looked like this:

- The father asked an informational question of the son.
- The son gave an evasive answer.
- The father became critical.
- The son put on sunglasses and fell silent.

Having made this observation, the therapist had the following exchange with the father:

Therapist: I wonder if you are finding out what you want to know?

Father: Well, not everything, but then some of it he may not know himself. So . . . I don't know . . . probably, yes.

Therapist: I don't think this is what you want, 'cause you really sound critical of him. You criticize him, and so he shuts up.

Father: (Pulls out hanky, blows his nose, glances at therapist, and lowers his eyes.)

Regardless of whether the content of this message was correct or not, an isomorphic transformation occurred that nullified it. The therapist played the role of the father, and the father took the role of his son:

- The therapist asked an informational question of the father.
- The father gave an evasive answer.
- The therapist became critical.
- The father pulled out a hanky and fell silent.

Although there were different participants, the outcome of each sequence was identical; one was a structural equivalent of the other.

It is this equivalence, this isomorphism that must be interrupted if change is to occur. The presence of isomorphic transformations is potentially a great help, since exposing just one of them can reverberate throughout the system, even affecting the larger versions that occur outside the interview room. Although hard to spot, they occur so often that therapists should not worry about eventually seeing them; as structuralists often observe, it is only the linear train that never goes around again.

Chapter 4 described a critical sequence in the Fletcher family, whereby Judy's slight movements away from her mother were followed by her brother's symptomatic behaviors. These, in turn, prompted the mother's protective stance toward Judy and in this way renewed their alliance as they teamed up against the "symptom bearer." Such sequences are in general quite concrete. They involve both verbal and nonverbal actions, and they occur in an almost casual way. Naturally, they are hard to notice because the therapist is so close to them. Therapists should not expect to "see" them until after several hours of interviewing. These sequences consist of at least three steps and generally more; any fewer reduces the therapist's chances to intervene successfully.

The Stone Family

A more detailed example of these small, on-the-spot sequences is provided by the Stone family, who came to treatment because the younger of their two children—a daughter, age 12—created long periods of selective silence. Although she would talk when away from home, as soon as she crossed the threshold from outside to inside the family she fell silent, consistently avoiding any communication with her father and exchanging only a few words with her mother, to whom she nonetheless physically clung in a regressed manner. From both observation and family report, anyone would assume that there was a cross-generational alliance between Mrs. Stone and her daughter; yet the Stones presented themselves as a perfectly amiable couple with no outstanding difficulties between them. The overriding purpose of this family resided almost entirely in their management of affect and of the family's appearance to the outer world. Their goal was to give the appearance of closeness, but without any meaningful emotional contact. The daughter's symptoms were an elegant parody of this—physically clinging to the mother while steadfastly refusing to say anything meaningful.

In the interview, the couple were cooperative and pleasant. To test their claim of parental accord, the therapist frequently directed them to discuss their daughter's problem without reference to her, although she was actually sitting between them. These discussions began efficiently but, within minutes, would end in disarray, leaving the therapeutic unit depleted. It was not apparent what had happened. Here is an excerpt from a typical interview:

Therapist: (Speaking to the parents) It will be helpful if the two of you discuss the things you've tried with this problem, Then I'll be able to catch up with your ideas. Let's hear what you think is going on here.

Father: (Looking at his wife) It's been this way for some time now. When did it start, dear, these long silences?

Mother: (Looking back at her husband) Since . . . oh, perhaps when she had the dog frighten her. But there's got to be more than that. It just angers me so, these unbelievable silences and then. . . .

Father: And then your sense of being accused of something. . . .

Mother: Yes! But you don't even really appreciate how it makes one feel, especially as a mother, I mean.

Daughter: (She is slumped in her chair, face and eyes down, staring at the floor. She quickly and briefly raises her head, looks directly at her mother with a pleading expression, and then lowers her head again.)

Father: You may be too upset about. . . .

Mother: No, no, no. You may be too calm about it. You need the full picture of how she hangs around me, saying nothing. (The mother now sounds angry.)

Father: (Shifting in his chair slightly so that he can now look at his daughter) I know it's a lot, but just calm down a bit. . . .

Mother: No! It gets to be too much. (She continues for a minute or so. Her husband no longer is responding to her.)

Father: (He remains quiet, calm in appearance, no longer engaged with his wife. He looks occasionally at his daughter, who continues to slump in her chair with eyes lowered.)

Mother: (She also now falls silent.)

Daughter: (She sits up a bit, shifts to a more comfortable position, but continues to remain silent.)

Father: I think she is sensitive about this (unclear as to which "she").

Therapist: (Speaking to the daughter) What about it, Lisa, why don't you tell them now what you think. Now's your chance. (The daughter remains silent.)

Close analysis of the videotapes revealed the following sequence, observed to occur as many as seven times in a single interview.

1. Following the therapist's instruction, *the mother and father looked at each other* and discussed their daughter's silence.
2. The daughter, who sat slumped in her chair with her head lowered, briefly, for no more than an instant, raised her head and *presented her face to her mother.* With a pleading expression, the daughter then quickly lowered her head.
3. The mother continued her chat with her husband, but now raised her voice angrily, complaining to him about the way her daughter *clung to her.* Her voice continued to rise.
4. The father then *broke eye contact* with his wife, turned slightly in his chair toward the daughter, and regarded her with concern. He did not silence his wife, but he stopped making verbal responses to her remarks.

5. The wife finally *fell silent*; the daughter visibly shifted to a more comfortable position in her chair; and the father continued to rest his eyes on her.
6. Silence reigned in the interview room.

Contrary to an earlier assumption, the cross-generational alliance that seemed to exist on this microcosmic level was that of the father and daughter against the mother. With virtually no words, this group succeeded in defeating the novelty of a parental coalition by rearranging itself into the more customary dyad of father and daughter. Therapy with this family seldom progressed beyond this point, because there were two further steps in the sequence:

7. In the silence that prevailed, the father finally shifted his eyes from his daughter to the therapist, signaling that "this" (i.e., silence) was the problem to be treated.
8. The therapist then began to talk to the daughter, trying to elicit some response from her. This effort implicitly sanctioned the split between the parents, giving the impression that the expert would handle the problem. But the power of this sequence always defeated the therapist.

CHANGING A SEQUENCE

When sequences have been located, how are they to be changed? First, the therapist privately arranges the sequence into several steps, listing them in the order of appearance. For the purposes of intervention, they should also be listed as though they occurred in a purely linear progression. While the underlying model continues to be one of circular causality, the therapist, as Gurman (1981) has pointed out, ". . . may choose to *punctuate* a long string of interactions in this way for purposes of intervention" (p. 316). Through such punctuation, certain events become primary targets for the therapist, even though, in the circular model, they have no more determining power in the sequence than any other event. The advantage of this linear pretense is to allow the therapist some option as to who in the family system might most successfully be involved in interrupting the sequence. That is, which step in the sequence becomes a focus for change depends in part on the therapeutic alliances at that moment, on the larger restructuring changes desired, and on some evaluation of the family's overall resistance to exposure of its principal secrets. By conceptualizing a circular chain as a sequence involving a discrete number of steps, the therapist then has the latitude to highlight, through punctuation, the step and the family players most likely to lend themselves to change. From this perspective, the therapist may use any of the following techniques to interrupt a sequence.

Describing and Instructing

The therapist "notices aloud" a critical aspect of the sequence and then joins this with a simple task assignment. The task is usually to continue a healthy coalition or to discontinue a cross-generational coalition that is troublesome. Whenever therapists choose to announce what they have noticed, they should conclude with a suggestion about how to continue the interaction. This suggestion has the status of a task assignment and should show regard for each of the family members. In the case of the Stone family, the therapist might say this:

Therapist: (Speaking directly to the wife, immediately after step 4 when her husband breaks eye contact with her) I notice your husband is now looking at your daughter, perhaps concerned for her, and has stopped looking at you. Ask him to continue speaking with you so that you two don't get sidetracked, and so your daughter can really understand how angry you are.

Assuming that this intervention fails, the mother may respond in a way that refuses an affiliation with the therapist.

Mother: I was finished anyway (said to the therapist). And I worry if she thinks I'm angry at her, because I'm really not. We are just concerned about her.

Here the mother blocks the therapist and implies a continued coalition with her husband ("We are just concerned . . . "), as though contact with him had not, in fact, been broken. If the therapist decides to continue this type of intervention, then another member of the family must be approached. In this instance, only the father remains, since it would be premature to challenge the silent daughter. The therapist could try this alternative.

Therapist: (Speaking directly to the father, following step 4) I notice your listening to your wife is interrupted by your concern for your daughter. This may give your wife the impression that you are not listening to her. So it would be helpful, now, for you and your wife to go on together, since she needs to say how angry she is. And since it's not really all clear, she (indicating the daughter) can listen and learn and speak up if she disagrees.

In addition to the simple description of the sequence step, the therapist here implies that the father would be naturally eager to convey to his daughter what he and his wife have maintained all along—namely, that there is no marital disharmony and that he and his wife are always able to work together. The therapist's instruction assumes this to be true and simply asks the husband to demonstrate it by continuing the conversation with his wife. The daughter is included and defined as either a silent learner or a vocal protester. Such descriptions and instructions may continue until the sequence is disrupted and the disequilibrium necessary for change is established.

As with the ushering in of all new information, comments about sequence will lead to change only if one is simultaneously restructuring the family system. Earlier, in Chapter 5, an excerpt from an interview with the Alfred family was presented to illustrate the redefinition of a presenting problem. There, the son was assaulting his stepfather at home and required frequent hospitalizations. During the interview, a sequence began to unfold which, if allowed to run its usual course, would have ended with the son physically striking his stepfather. Just prior to that step, the therapist interrupted the flow and offered a detailed description of what was happening:

Therapist: (Looking at the stepfather) Just hold on. (Then moving to the chair next to the son and addressing his comments to him) I'll give you an idea of how you got into this fight . . . I'll tell ya how you got into this fight . . . you do when your mother says she's helpless. When your mother indicates that she's trapped . . . , and she can't do anything. You get pulled into fighting at this time.

The point here is not just the accuracy of the sequence description. The point is that it was *structurally* correct to address the remarks to the son. In this way, the therapist directly treated the son as a potential bystander to the conflict, rather than as a primary participant, and indirectly let the mother and stepfather become bystanders as they overheard the therapist's comments. Had the therapist addressed his remarks about the mother *to* the mother, he would have simply occupied the stepfather's place as her attacker, an ironic and isomorphic transformation of the very scenario that he was describing. In that position, he would of course have been attacked by the son, who would thereby have lost any chance of making an alliance with the one person, the therapist, who could have offered him a way out of the system. The sequence will change when an accurate description is offered in a way that also restructures the dysfunctional system.

Task Assignments

The alternative to description is to leave aside one's "noticings" and to proceed with straightforward task assignments. This may be the preference of therapists who put little reliance on the potency of verbal explanations and opt instead for more directed behavior change. A particularly critical task often assigned in sequence disruption is the blocking of a cross-generational alliance that has the status of a coalition against a third person. Such tasks, framed as briefly as possible, omit detailed descriptions or inferences about what people may be feeling. In the Stone family, the therapist may notice the crucial steps in the family's sequence and then assign the following task:

> *Therapist:* (Speaking to the mother and father) Your talking together is good, even about being angry. You should help your daughter by continuing this for another five minutes. Just look at each other, and say all you have to say about feeling angry. Her job (indicating the daughter) will be to be quiet and not distract you.

In this instance, the therapist briefly praises the parents, directs them to do even more with each other, and prescribes for the daughter a behavior (silence) that she is already practicing. The task has a time limit, some cues about nonverbal behavior ("look at each other"), and a definite theme (talking about anger). Other rules for task setting will be reviewed in Chapter 7.

Paradoxical Reframing

This is not a technique specifically derived from structural family therapy, but it is widely used to achieve the system's disequilibrium needed before the family can move to a better arrangment of its organization. In the Stone family, the therapist could make this comment:

> *Therapist:* (Speaking to the daughter following the completion of step 5) This silence is wonderful and helpful, and you are to be congratulated for knowing how to bring it about, for knowing that your father and mother prefer this to any angry exchanges *between themselves.* You understand how upset they get with anger, so you always signal them, especially your father, that *you* are getting upset. This helps them become concerned about you rather than angry at each other. That is a good outcome in a family that values closeness and harmony. Keep up the good work.

This comment is an ironic phrasing of a likely hypothesis. The irony is in the apparent support of the daughter's continuing her symptom, something she is bound to do until her parents (1) coalesce together into a well-bounded parenting system and (2) show a capacity for conflict. The family will either respond with utter opposition and disbelief, in which case the therapist is entitled to expect them to behave in accordance with their ideals—namely, that they cooperate together and are not intolerant of conflict. Or the family may feel relieved that the game is up and can now position themselves for change. Paradox is such a complicated phenomena that this discussion can only briefly indicate its usefulness in structural therapy. There have by now been many volumes written about paradox and strategic therapy, and readers should consult those works before venturing too far into this area. (See especially the work of Madanes, 1980; Palazzoli, 1978; and Papp, 1981.)

Using Sequence Analysis

One may use the formalities of a sequence analysis to focus on those themes of human experience that the therapist, generally on the basis of some a priori basis, happens to believe are most crucial to life. In this way, for example, a therapist who believes there is no change without a significant focus on the family's affect can retain the belief but be substantially aided by analyzing the repetitive ways in which feelings are handled. We may speak of the competent or incompetent handling of affect [if we wish to follow the competence model provided by Haley (1976)], noting what happens when someone in the family makes a new move to respond competently to the affective aspect of some event. Similarly, therapists interested in *learning styles* and *information processing* in the family can nonetheless benefit from a sequential analysis of what happens to, for example, an informational bit that is dropped into the family's communication network. Any special therapeutic interest may be followed as long as it is regarded as the content, which must first be regarded from the structural perspective that observes how it sequentially flows through the system.

SUMMARY

Description and instruction, task assignment, and paradoxical reframing are standard techniques for altering dysfunctional sequences. When combined with a consistent attention to the structure of family process, rather than to the thematic content, the structural family therapist is positioned to help the family change. Finally, the staging of these interventions and the notion of a treatment process that occurs in stages will assist the therapist in slowing down the flow of interactional material that, at first glance, makes the process of change seem so awesome. In the next chapter, the classic interventions of behavioral description and task assignment, already introduced in connection with sequence disruption, will be explored more deeply.

Chapter 7

Classic Interventions: Tasks and Descriptions

Assignments to engage in behavioral exchanges, either at home or in the interview, are commonplace interventions in structural family therapy. Tasks are the logical continuation of the emphasis on observed rather than reported behavior, of the therapist's position as leader of the therapeutic effort, and of the theoretical assumption that systems need to be challenged by creating new interactional sequences. A good task that is successfully assigned and completed signals that the therapeutic system is operating with a structural diagnosis and a plan for change that has effectively engaged all the family players. Tasks that fail or are poorly assigned, on the other hand, provide helpful opportunities, even mandates, for a refinement of the diagnosis and of the treatment plan.

Structuralists assume tasks are integral to change. Tasks, it is believed, more clearly lead to change than do descriptions; yet, in one form or another, offering explanations and promoting insight and other ways of telling a family the hows and whys of its life are present throughout the therapeutic process. Whether directly or indirectly, with or without theoretical rationale, therapists continue to tell people about their behavior. In this chapter, both task assignment and behavioral description are examined as intervention strategies.

THE TASKS OF CHANGE

All psychotherapy is directive, but some forms are more openly so than are others. This must be the case, since all therapists try to influence behavior. Although one might hope that individuals are destined to be whole and self-repairing, a less innocent and more deterministic model of development assumes that things often go wrong that are correctable by the creation of another "growing environment," whether that of the interpersonal-analytic context or that of the family interactional context. In any but the most nativist view of life, all models of change involve some degree of directiveness. Whether or not this becomes a trademark of any particular therapy's philosophy depends on several factors, one of which is candidness.

Most practitioners of structural family therapy are openly directive of the change process, although through circularity they are also followers of the family's poorly formed, but nonetheless existing, wishes for change. This capacity to be formed by the family, as well as to form it, needs emphasis before one learns all about giving directives, tasks, and so forth. Too frequently, the active therapist views the family as an essentially resistant body with no sense of how life should move ahead. From such a perspective, the therapist seems to act upon the family, directing change in an almost linear way. Closer analysis (e.g., Umbarger & Bernstein, 1979) shows a more circular model of therapeutic interaction, with *the family frequently providing the cues* for new directions. The competent therapist follows these cues, articulates them into states of greater clarity, and then retires to let the family continue at its own pace. To follow respectfully as well as to lead actively offers therapists the balance they need to feel comfortable in offering directives.

Who Sets Tasks?

Two groups of therapists set tasks. These groups differ in the degrees of openness with which they make assignments. One is a group of "indirect directors" such as hypnotists and most psychoanalytic psychotherapists. Hypnotists, particularly those influenced by Milton Erikson, may become masters of covert induction into trance. And many analytic therapists offer directions while denying that they are doing so, as in the instruction to "do nothing" except to have "free associations," a rather considerable and probably paradoxical request despite the emphasis on "doing nothing." Many other therapists attempt to influence the internal imagery of clients by emphasizing to them specific "critical" episodes in their past life and asking for "spontaneous" associations to such events. A second group of task assigners are more explicitly directive. This group includes most family therapists (except those involved in paradoxical interventions) and most behaviorists. There is no special morality in being either more or less open about one's degree of directiveness as long as such activity is consistent with the metatheory that guides the interventions and is designed for the welfare of the client.

Why Does One Set Tasks?

With few exceptions, tasks can speed up both the diagnostic and the therapeutic process, involving people in new routines of behavior that encourage change. Below are some frequent reasons for task assignment.

To Observe Symptomatic Behavior

To observe the symptomatic behavior in the interview room is often better than simply to hear about it—unless the symptom is physically dangerous or deeply humiliating. Most issues of child management and many instances of psychotic communication can best be observed if the family is directed to demonstrate, in the safety of the interview room, those interpersonal sequences that usually contain the symptom. This demonstration gives the therapist excellent diagnostic information and a chance to feel sympathetic with the true dimensions of the family's struggle.

EXAMPLE. An overburdened single mother complained that her oldest daughter, age seven, was persistently defiant and stubborn, while her two younger daughters were easy to manage. In the interview, the index daughter was polite and responsive to the therapist and only mildly impersonal to her mother. The therapist arranged for the three children to begin playing with blocks and using the art easel while the mother gave some personal views of the problem. After about 15 minutes, the therapist instructed the mother to ask her children to put away the blocks and paints. She and her oldest daughter plunged rapidly into a struggle that threatened to escalate to physical dimensions. The "good" children were observed to snicker and show mild amusement at their mother's ineffective efforts, an irritant that made the mother even more angry at her defiant daughter. When the daughter threatened to scribble on the office walls with felt tip markers, the therapist joined the mother in physically restraining her. As the daughter wept and raged, the mother was visibly relieved to find the therapist in the same boat with her. Seconds later, she spoke sharply to the other daughters, telling them that they were not to laugh, that this was a serious matter, and that they should be careful of their older sister's feelings. In this event, the therapist not only saw when the symptom occurred, but also discovered that the mother could act competently to protect this vulnerable child even while angry at her.

To Observe Latent Conflict

To expose latent conflict in the family may be considered impolite by some, but is often helpful, especially when a scapegoating process is occurring. Minuchin (1974) described a group of parents who regularly detoured their own conflicts through one child, often allowing the other children to join in. When such a situation arises, it is helpful to introduce to the family a more complex viewpoint by showing that there are several factors involved in the "family problem" and that no single factor alone is responsible for the family's difficulties. The task assigned should help the latent conflict to surface, thereby eroding the rigid focus on the index child and should, in this way, detriangulate the child from the parental dyad.

In confronting this generic problem (the agreeable couple whose life is marred only by a single difficult child), the structural therapist will usually assign a task. Since invariably, one of the parents is, by agreement, the active manager of this child, a standard task is to request the parent who is peripheral to apply management skills actively to the child and to support the *public* stance that the parenting behavior of each spouse is the same. After a few days of this new regime, concealed differences between the parents usually appear. This happens because the peripheral parent nearly always has secret sympathies with the scapegoated child, sympathies that show up during the management efforts. The other spouse, now excluded by the task, will become critical during this arrangement. The covert differences now become visible to all and easier to address. The detouring of conflict is no longer possible.

To Establish New Alliances

To establish new alliances is probably the most familiar goal of task assignments. In one way it is a wonderfully direct approach to the problem of weak affiliations. When mothers and daughters or fathers and sons have no tie to each other, the therapist simply designs a situation where they may begin to build up a history of shared experiences. There may be suggestions for weekend ventures, bedtime stories, shopping trips or special projects. Such tasks must be carefully designed but are straightforward in their intentions. In examples drawn from the Fletcher family it would be obvious to assign some tasks to the father and his two sons. Other issues may be addressed besides that of new affiliations, as in the following example.

EXAMPLE. The Darcy family, as mentioned in Chapter 6, consisted of the parents, both alcoholic and in their mid-50s, a son, age 30 and alcoholic, and another son, age 21, who was schizophrenic. They all lived at home. The only social contact was between Mrs. Darcy and the youngest son. She supervised everything from his meals to his bowel movements. There was minimal contact between the parents or between either parent and the older son. This family had many complaints, a frequent one being that John, the older son, came home drunk in the early morning hours, without his house-key. He would pound on the front door until the parents awoke and let him in. During the evening hours, while John was out, the parents drank in separate rooms, the mother accompanied by her younger son. The therapist assigned the following task: Mr. Darcy and John were to spend three nights a week at the father's favorite local tavern. They were free to drink as much as they liked, but they were to come home together, using the father's house-key. They were to talk about sports and other current events, finding out what the other liked. This task was designed to do three things: (1) to break the rule that only the mother was to have close alliances and that the father and John were not; (2) to solve the problem of John coming home in a disruptive manner; and (3) to begin to address the issues of alcohol abuse. Naturally, this task would promote only a temporary stage in the treatment, since nothing was included about Mrs. Darcy's overinvolvement with the other son nor was the marital unit involved.

To Establish Therapeutic Rule Breaking

To establish therapeutic rule breaking as an open and acceptable routine in the family, a therapist may request the family to practice certain unfamiliar actions. All families have routines of behavior that de facto make up their "rules" for living. Therapists need to help the family challenge troublesome rules by practicing new behaviors. For example, in a family in which a dyadic fight is allowed to involve all family members, the family might be requested to have two days in which that "rule" is set aside and a new one tried—namely, that the two people who are in a fight band together angrily to oppose any other family member who wants to get in on it. This intervention serves not only to set up a new rule, one that permits dyads some integrity, but may even soften the fight between the two principals.

EXAMPLE. When following up on the task assigned to the Darcys, the therapist found that they had not carried it out, principally due to an overriding family rule that read, "Cooperation is for suckers; broken promises make good protection." The therapist responded to the Darcys' broken promise (to do the task) in the following manner:

Therapist: In your home, it is usual for people to promise things and then not follow through, for whatever reason. Nobody cooperates with anybody. But here, in my "home," my office, there are different ground rules, and I want to practice them. I'm breaking your rule. This interview is over . . . don't even bother to sit down. Go home and practice breaking your rule instead of breaking your promises. When your promise to me is kept and you have been drinking together, call me and we will have another meeting.

The therapist then left the room amid startled and angry comments from the family. The Darcys were then able to practice "rule breaking" and to resume their therapy.

To Develop Behavior Management Strategies

To develop new strategies in behavior management, many therapists join with parents in designing tasks that will allow them to practice alternative responses to the presenting problem.

EXAMPLE. The Finemans were a warm and humorous group. The parents were loving toward each other and toward their two sons. Joel, age 18, was an excellent student and athlete. David, age 12, was also an excellent student, but socially immature. David concerned his parents because he seemed clinging, easily tearful, kept secrets (the mother's special concern), and was given to temper outbursts. When these behaviors were absent, David was cheerful and cooperative. His parents were especially angry about his early morning behavior: David would not get out of bed until both parents had made separate efforts to rouse him. He complained of vague aches and ills, would finally get up only after an angry exchange with his cajoling parents, and after a sloppy job of dressing, would barely make it to school on time. In school he was well liked and did excellent work. In consultation with the parents, the therapist discovered that Mrs. Fineman always enjoyed waking David, ever since he was quite small. David had never had his own alarm clock nor had the parents ever considered it.

His issues with sleep were not, however, confined to waking up, but also extended to going to sleep. At night, he made frequent trips to his parents' bedroom after they had retired to watch TV or read. Often David would make his last visit to them around midnight. The parents and the therapist decided to try a new strategy for David's sleeping and waking problems, something other than indulgence or shouting. Since the issues around night-time separations seemed especially loaded, they decided to address his waking up. The parents bought David an alarm clock and told him that he was now to wake himself, although his mother would continue to have breakfast ready for him and would make sure there were clean clothes. David could elect to stay in bed, and his parents agreed that if he missed school there would be no punishments. Being in school was his business. They also mentioned that they would be leaving the house together every morning just a few minutes before 7:45, a reasonable time for boys to leave for school. The parents had decided to spend some of those mornings having a special, second cup of coffee at their favorite restaurant before each went to work. David was dismayed and filled with aches. He missed school for the first two days. He refused to set his alarm clock. The parents phoned the therapist, were reassured, and then resumed a firm, but kindly position with David. They refrained from shouting. This new strategy eventually succeeded, no doubt in part because of David's healthy interest in being in school where he performed so well. His nighttime problems diminished considerably, as he felt he needed more sleep if he was to get himself up when his alarm went off.

To Empower New Family Subsystems

To empower new family subsystems, one may devise tasks that provide an opportunity for cooperation and affiliation that were previously absent. Such moves, because they are directed at establishing the power and boundary integrity of some normal subunit, involve more than establishing new alliances. The most common example is a task that requires the marital unit to become more prominent and well bounded. This kind of task may include, for instance, sending the parents away for a weekend together or simply arranging with the children to allow some part of each evening during which they will not interrupt their parents. Below is an example of empowering the sibling unit.

EXAMPLE. Mr. and Mrs. Wayne had been married for two years. It was a second marriage for both of them, and each brought children into the marriage. The parents were highly intellectual and introspective and were determined that their second marriage would be successful. Both seemed annoyed by the presence of their children, three girls and two boys, ranging in age from 12–18. Two of the children were symptomatic. Mr. Wayne's oldest daughter, 18, was recovering from a serious episode of depression that had required her hospitalization. She was now ready to leave a halfway house and return to the family home. Mrs. Wayne's youngest child, a 12-year-old boy, was encopretic, socially immature, and overweight. The remaining three children were doing well in school and at home. Efforts to activate the parents into greater concern about the children were not going well. The household was in great disarray: rooms were dirty; there was seldom enough to eat; there was no supervision of either waking or bedtime hours; and the parents simply stayed away from the house many evenings. Not only was the household disorganized, but little progress had been made in uniting the children of these recently married parents. While there was no open fighting, there was no cooperation either. Faced with the resistance of the parental unit, the imminent return of the depressed daughter, and the continued soiling by the son, the therapist got permission from the parents to meet alone with the five children. After a single preliminary meeting, the therapist assigned a task: the children were to form a kind of tribal council, including the daughter about to return home, and were to devise rules for running the household. They were to return next week and meet with the therapist for further planning. The children did even more. They organized an overnight camping trip to one of the city's large parks. There, they had an evening meeting around a campfire and, managing to escape harassment by locals and arrest by the police, actually drew up a rather complicated series of decrees that covered both domestic and psychological matters. The therapist, with continued parental permission, met with this group of siblings for six weeks until they formed a lobby with enough internal definition and enough unit strength to force the parents into at least partial participation in family life.

What Types of Tasks Are There?

Typologies usually reduce complex phenomena to such simplistic states that the resulting concepts have all the sophistication of bumper stickers. Nonetheless, in discussing task assignments students repeatedly raise two questions that lend themselves to some form of typology. The first question is invariably about the degree of awareness clients should have about the intention of the task: do they knowingly participate or is some covert manipulation involved? The second question is quite pragmatic: when does one assign them? This is literally a concern with a purely temporal dimension and concerns whether one assigns a task now, in the office, perhaps, or as an activity to be carried out at some later date. In terms of the dimension of a client's relative awareness, types of tasks may be generally distributed in this way:

UNAWARE	SOMEWHAT AWARE	MOSTLY AWARE
Indirect hypnosis	Analytic interpretation	Behavior modification
Tricks	Tasks	Tasks
Paradox		

Only at the *Unaware* end of the continuum might one argue that clients are not direct participants in the change process, and even there, proponents of paradoxical prescription, for instance, could point out the family's intuitive sense of what is going on. *Tasks* are listed under both of the other two continuum points since they may, depending on one's intention, be made more or less clear. In one regard, the family is always a willing participant in carrying out tasks since it must agree with the rationale offered by the therapist when the task is proposed. That is, one needs to "frame" the task so that family members agree to carry it out; in this spirit, one can assume that the family is generally aware of the probable thrust of the task. Only when a family consistently misuses explanation and openness to continue its opposition to change might a therapist cloak task assignments in vague or elusive language. In those instances, the therapist helps the family avoid its own oppositional tendencies by mentioning that the task will be "interesting for those who want to prove their point," or will "help some of you in the way you want, but not all of you," or may be "just the thing to do the trick," without specifying what that "trick" is. In all these elusive phrasings, one might suspect that the family is "somewhat aware" of the task's aim, but the full intentions are not pointedly discussed between therapist and family.

There are several types of tasks that beginning therapists are tempted to use, but should avoid. One is a simple assignment to change, usually involving a kind of "thought stoppage." Here you find therapists who tell someone that "For the next week, you are not to let Jimmy wet his bed, tease the hamster, or split his infinitives, or engage in whatever symptom bothers you." This requirement for direct change seldom works. Second, tasks are sometimes used as a "last resort," even as a kind of punishment for the recalcitrant family. These assignments generally embarrass people and are not really designed to succeed as much as to get power back for the therapist. Such therapists will use the family's failure as proof of its need to be in therapy. Finally, there are tasks that are well intentioned but naively thought through, as in the assignment of "ordeal" tasks to utterly compliant families. This is a variation of the "punishment" task, though the therapist is truly innocent of ill intentions, and the task generally involves an element of paradox. Such families resist the change via paradox and simply suffer the outrage. For example, asking this kind of family to address its chronic problem of household dirt and general mess by leaving garbage in the living room only results in a dirtier house.

In addition to degree of "client consciousness," one may classify types of tasks according to *when* in the course of treatment a therapist assigns a task. This is a matter of timing and of therapist control. If the task is to be completed during the interview, the therapist has more control over its course than if the task is to be carried out in the client's home. Typing according to timing and degree of therapist presence looks like this:

IN IMAGINATION	ACTION NOW	AT HOME
Just imagine moving across this room to sit next to your mother.	Please say that to your ____________ right now, here.	Tonight let your husband put Billy to bed while you relax.

By far the most frequent tasks used in structural therapy are those that occur during the interview. In a sense, most restructuring interventions have the status of task assignments inasmuch as they frequently request people to behave differently. Structural therapists ask people to do things in the interview; when these requests are properly framed, they constitute a task given to the family. Observe these examples:

Therapist: Now, Mrs. N., since you don't need your daughter's help when speaking with your husband, please keep her from interrupting for the next five minutes while you go on.

• • • •

It would be easier for the two of you to sit together while talking. So would you and [whoever] please switch chairs.

• • • •

In this family where everyone is concerned about everybody else, all your business gets mixed up. And you speak for each other. For the next ten minutes, everyone gets to finish the sentence that he or she starts, and no one is to interrupt.

• • • •

Your son makes those noises and grimaces, the ones he was doing in the hospital, when your wife gets upset. You and your wife should continue talking, but I want you to sit next to him and touch him lightly on the arm if he starts those things. You are to reassure him and help him manage better.

These examples of directives are common enough to structural therapists, but may be uncomfortable, even offensive to therapists trained in tactics of noninterference. There are often excellent reasons for letting a family's process develop naturally during the interview, especially at the beginning. It is also apparent that many therapists are resistant to being directive, not because of their theoretical orientation, but because of their personal resistances to the immediacy of feeling and action that their directives may evoke. In some ways, all people are afraid of emotion, especially moments of deep feelings, and would prefer to hear reports about feelings and conflict rather than to arrange circumstances that would provoke their direct occurrence in the interview setting among the major figures of the family drama. One's own personal issues are intensified whenever one moves authoritatively to evoke the forces of family conflict. To avoid this discomfort, therapists may cite (1) the rights of patients to move at their own pace; (2) the fear of being authoritarian or of manipulating others; and (3) some concerns about permanent change versus symptomatic relief (true "growth" rather than directed behavior change). The structural preference for direction is partially based on an assumption that clients are more open to change and at a more rapid rate than usually assumed. Furthermore, the evoking of feelings during the interview, as well as the designed practice of new behaviors, often adds credibility to the family's original complaints. Like a person taking a broken radio to the shop only to find that it works perfectly, families often feel foolish in their complaints, since there is no phenomenal evidence of the complaints during the interview: the children are beautifully behaved, the disturbed adolescent is suddenly free of voices, the unhappy husband is now fully content with his marriage, and so on. Directing people in the interview relieves them of the frustration of simply reporting about behavior and allows them to prove that the radio is really on the blink.

How Does One Set Tasks?

Even when therapists are clear as to why they wish to assign a task and when it should happen, there remains the delicate action of announcing it. One master of this is Braulio Montalvo, best seen in his film *A Family With a Little Fire* (Philadelphia Child Guidance Clinic Video Series; also, in Minuchin, 1974). A close review of that film shows all the critical steps in correct task assignment. Montalvo was confronted with a single-parent family, which was overburdened and poor, yet still close and struggling to move ahead. The oldest daughter, age seven, had set several fires at home, one of which might have been serious had it not been for the quick action of her older brother, a parental child who looked after his sibs when the mother was away. Near the end of the interview, Montalvo made a daring, but simple assignment: he asked the mother, angry as she was, to teach her daughter how to play with matches in a safe way. The intent of the task was to repair the alliance between the mother and daughter, to help the parental child be less active, and above all, to control the fire setting. The following is a useful guide for all task setting and is based on Montalvo's interview.

Assessing Family Mood

The emotional tone of Montalvo's task needed to match the family's mood in the interview moment. Montalvo sensed that the mother was ready for some reconciliation with her daughter and that her anger was about to change into concern. The emotional time was right. In general, if the task is to be fun, it should be assigned when the family's mood is lighter and more hopeful; if the task will be unsettling, perhaps exposing latent conflict, the mood must be serious. An assignment of the "let's-get-together-and-try-again" type, when the family's mood is one of utter despair, is doomed to fail.

Framing the Task

The therapist should offer a framework and rationale that are acceptable at least to the key members who will be involved. In Montalvo's case, he repeated several times to the mother that she had done a good job raising the daughter and that she must want to protect her to see that she didn't hurt herself with matches. At the same time, he told the daughter that learning how to play with matches safely would be a chance for her to show her mother what she knew about matches and, most importantly, that it would be a "game" which only she, of all the children, could play with mommy. In general, the rationale needs to make sense, and to have some bearing on the presenting problem and its elaboration. The correct framing will make it possible for some of the family members to agree to do it; an insufficient rationale will interest nobody, although out of politeness, the family may agree to carry it out, but then fail to do so.

Including Reluctant Members

In many ways, this is the most critical aspect of successful task setting. One's central structural hypothesis informs the selection of players. Montalvo recognized how much the parental child, a boy of 11, was involved as a go-between for the mother and daughter; hence, the task was directed not only at strengthening the alliance between the mother and daughter, but at giving a new role to the son. He mentioned all three of them by name, giving principal attention to the mother and daughter, but asking the son to stay out so he could have time to do parenting with the other, younger children. It was a simple, but essential move because Montalvo knew that no one involved in the problem may be omitted from the task. His task also showed that patterned behavior may be deflected from some specific object, but the behavior itself cannot simply be shut off. Thus, he deflected the parenting behavior of the son from the index patient so that the mother was allowed to move into alliance with her troubled daughter. He did not, however, expect the son to give up his parenting role altogether. Instead, he asked him to look after the younger children so that the mother and daughter would have time to do the task. Most tasks fail because the therapist has not included those family members most involved in perpetuating the problem. One does not simply disengage critical components of a structure by assigning them duties elsewhere. If, for example, a parent is overfunctioning or overly competent, one may wish to direct that away from the index patient, but the behavior of overfunctioning must be anchored elsewhere. In the Darcy family, cited above, the mother's overconcerned behavior with her son was deflected from him to a nearby nursing home where she was encouraged to do volunteer work three days a week. There, her overconcern became actually appropriate to the debilitated condition of the sick and elderly, while the son was freed to show more competence about matters of his personal hygiene. A good task has something of potential value for all who are involved in it.

Setting Time Limits

Tasks that are open-ended with regard to duration take on unhelpful moral tones, sounding like injunctions to "go forth and sin no more." Change is hard, and one only sustains a bit for a little while. Hence, a task should have time limits. Montalvo helped the mother accept the task by saying that she was only to help her daughter use matches two or three times in the next week and then for only five or ten minutes each trial. He advised her to use an egg timer and immediately stop the "play" if it stopped being fun. He permitted the mother and daughter to begin this new and problematic event by building in a time to stop it. The time limits of a task will vary with the degree of complexity, the number of players involved, and the activity itself. Sometimes the outer limit is a weekend, as when the parents arrange to take a trip by themselves. Other tasks require brief periods of time, often occurring at the same point in the day, as when a parent and child set aside designated time periods to find out about the day at school or simply to give special attention to a child excluded from parental favor. Permission for a clear ending will increase the chances of actually beginning the task.

Assessing the Outcome

In the second interview with the fire-setting family, Montalvo was confronted with a relieved and happy mother and a relaxed and happy daughter. The task had been carried out, and both participants had obviously enjoyed it. The parental child had also succeeded at his end of it. To follow up this success, Montalvo asked for a demonstration of the mother's teaching by suggesting that she help the daughter set a fire in a large ashtray. The mother did this, and the daughter succeeded in building a contained fire. The task had been helpful in allaying fears that things would get out of control. As Montalvo said to the mother, in a confident and reassuring voice, about her daughter's dexterity with matches: "The fingers now, they are working real nice." In making a follow-up of the task, therapists will discover either how the family cooperated to carry out the task or how it colluded to undermine it. Too frequently a therapist assumes a failed task reflects therapeutic inadequacy. Perhaps there was a fault in framing the rationale, or some other fault, but it is equally likely that the family conspired to defeat the changes inherent in the task. Only a detailed inquiry will show a therapist the parts of the structural puzzle that have been missed, the family member mistakenly thought not crucial to the problem, or the resistance of a parent that is more pervasive than one knew. The failure to follow up a task and to assess its fate in the family system rapidly undermines the credibility and power of a therapist; if, the family may wonder, the task was not worth inquiring about, was it worth assigning in the first place?

In summary, the assignment of behavioral tasks is an important strategy for change used by structural therapists. It provides concrete action around the particular behaviors judged essential in maintaining a dysfunctional system. Tasks are rapid avenues into deeper diagnostic pictures (particularly when a task fails) and into the development of new behavior routines. With few exceptions, tasks should be assigned with success in mind and for straightforward purposes. When tasks fail, the credibility of the therapist can be rescued by making a competent follow-up, thereby increasing the therapist's view of the family's complicated structural forces.

DESCRIPTION AND CHANGE

Whether or not people change their behavior because they learn to understand the contextual constraints on both their inner and their interpersonal life is an unanswered question. Those in favor of omitting explanations of behavior—the reasons "why" something happens—argue that there is no evidence to support the usefulness of insight. Nonetheless, people insist on acting as if they are rational creatures and hence persist in using explanation and understanding in most of their communicational exchanges, whether or not their therapist is in favor of it. The topic is delicate and speculative, since the behavioral sciences seem unlikely to resolve the matter one way or the other. Those therapists who believe that change comes through understanding the forces in family life will continue to tell the family many of their speculations; therapists who are wary of explanations will continue to provide alternative avenues for change, but must be ready to accept whatever explanations the family may insist on providing.

Minuchin and Fishman have themselves varied on this matter, commenting at one time that "Cognitive constructions per se are rarely powerful enough to spark family change" (1981, p.117). Yet throughout this same text, they often urged therapists to help the family change its reality and its world view by increased understanding of the behavioral options that therapists provide. The interventions of Minuchin and Fishman themselves often took the form of circular explanations: X does this, then Y responds, which further activates X, and so on. By assigning reciprocity and announcing to the family this circular model of cause and effect, they were asking the family to participate in a cognitive scheme about its own family experience. The emphasis always remains on interactive descriptions, on *how* behaviors are linked into interactive chains, and not on *why* this may be occurring. By avoiding speculations about motivation, the therapist frees the family from positions of blaming or of guilt and allows the family to appreciate the artful mechanics of its interlocked behaviors.

While the larger issue—is explanation helpful?—seems far from resolution, there is a pragmatic position that therapists may take. That position is to accept people's need to feel rational and hence capable of benefiting from knowing about themselves, and yet to offer such descriptions only with prior respect for new and healthier structural pathways that are the ultimate goal of therapy. Explanations and descriptions, no matter how psychologically accurate, are wasted if they are introduced through the structures that maintain family pathology. In this way, the issue is not so much the presence or absence of understanding, but to whom in the family, and in what way, such information is offered. For example, in the case of Ken, the boy who was attacking his stepfather (Chapter 5), the therapist offered an explanation about how fighting started in the family. The explanation may or may not have been correct, but the *structurally* correct part of that intervention was that the explanation was given to the disturbed son, a move consistent with the therapist's effort to create a bystander role for the son, thereby removing him from his role as one of the mother's enmeshed champions. From this pragmatic position, structural therapists use a number of "strategies for telling" in their efforts to change families.

Therapist as Expert

Therapists occasionally must offer expert testimony to families in order to impress upon them the gravity of outcomes they are denying. In some families, the collective capacity for reality testing has become so shredded through the progressive breakdown of mechanisms for collecting and assessing information that an outsider, in this case the therapist, must perform that service for them. Families with seriously ill children, homicidal episodes, or repeated psychotic behaviors often require persistent reminders about the behavioral sequences that typically lead to such eruptions. In those instances, the therapist must forcefully take the lead and correct the family's *laissez-faire* attitude. Not to do so would most probably lead to another harmful symptomatic outburst.

In the role of expert, a therapist may also draw on accumulated clinical evidence to support predictions about future outcomes. For example, when the last child in a family has, due to a psychotic episode, been forced to return home after only a short time away at college, any therapist who arrives on the case early enough may challenge moments of family denial by saying: "This child will be with you for many years, perhaps until you die, unless we can confront the problem immediately." In essence, the therapist says, "This is a well-known family event, the clinical outcome of which is a pathological arrangement for keeping the child at home forever." The delivery of expert testimony may be done calmly, but with the firm force of clinical conviction and experience.

Therapist as Educator

A step away from the expert's role is that of educational instructor. There are many instances in which dysfunctional behavioral sequences occur through ignorance, not through malevolence. Parents and children are often quite open to learning through the educational inputs of the therapist. Some mothers with young children, fathers with no parenting models, immigrants to a new setting, and upwardly mobile ethnic families may be in need of simple educational instructions, including the assignment of books. An educational approach not only assumes the best about people, but may provide an oblique and polite way out of potentially awkward situations. In one family, for example, the adolescent daughter was hospitalized at a prestigious retreat following her arrest on prostitution charges and a subsequent psychotic episode. Her father, though he had been in this country for many years, still retained distinct features of his ethnic origins. During visits to the hospital, the father would hold the daughter on his lap, groom her hair, kiss her, and behave in ways the staff found upsetting. The daughter reciprocated these overtures. Hesitant to do anything, the chief resident called on an outside consultant, who advised the staff to consider this a matter of cultural misunderstanding and thus one that could be corrected by educational instruction. The staff was to announce to the father the following: "We must tell you, to avoid any further misunderstanding, that here in America fathers and daughters of her age do not do these things. We discussed it and were sure you would want to know this thing." This stopped the father's provocative behavior. Regardless of underlying family issues, treating the event as a cultural misunderstanding permitted an educational intervention. Many clients would like to change their behavior, but cannot think of a face-saving way to do so; the use of educational instruction gives them that opportunity.

Therapist as Describer

Another technique of description has already been mentioned—that of sequence description. This is probably the most common form of telling people about themselves. It supplies the links in a circular dance, tells all participants about the roles they characteristically play, and explains how this dance then becomes troublesome. Any description of a behavioral transaction—whether a six-step sequence among many family members or a brief dyadic exchange—falls into this category of explanation. As with all instances of telling, the therapist must pay close attention not just to the truth of the comment, but to how it is received by the family and whether or not it makes any impact. A good sequence description should have the status of a task assignment. That is, a successful description requires the therapist to assess the mood of the family, timing, who is to be included in the description, and so forth; when the system is attentive and open to new information, then a sequence description can be most helpful.

Just this side of traditional interpretation is a type of telling that is a kind of *guided revelation,* an engineered exercise in discovering patterns of behavior that the therapist has already observed or intuits are present. Some task assignments are intended to achieve such revelations, showing family members the aspects of their structured experience that were previously concealed from them or revealing opportunities for new experiences that were only dimly imagined. Family sculpture techniques are the best examples of guided revelation, since every spatial rearrangement is accompanied by new learning on the part of the participants and extensive commentary by the therapist-guide. This type of telling differs from simple sequence description (which is the recounting of behaviors occurring spontaneously) through the intentional design of experiences that, when completed, should yield new ideas about the family process of living together.

Therapist as Interpreter

Far removed from the techniques of expert testimony or educational instruction is traditional interpretation. On the basis of observations and many a priori assumptions about intrapsychic process, the therapist offers explanations about the family problem. These ideas concern inner motivations, feeling states attributed to individual members, and the provision of psychodynamic linkages between transactional behavior and inner psychological states. The intention is to promote insight into the reasons why people behave as they do and to suggest that certain public behaviors are inevitable, given the presence of private, internal forces. This form of telling involves theoretical constructs that lie wholly outside a systems paradigm of behavior, but that are often congenial to clients well versed in traditional dynamic psychology. When interpretative procedures are congruent with the family's style of changing, they may be used by a structural therapist, but always with preeminent regard for the impact on underlying patterns of alliance and structural function.

Therapist as Reframer

Throughout all techniques for telling and explaining, one constant feature is that of positive reframing. Although not obviously derived from the theory of structural family therapy, reframing is everywhere used in the clinical application of structural principles. For that reason, it merits a special place as an explanatory intervention.

To reframe something is simply to attend to a *different* facet of the multifaceted reality of any particular behavior. In a pluralistic and perspectivistic universe, what something is depends in large part on when one views it and from what point in the system. If, for example, Mr. Fletcher's low rate of behavioral exchange with his children seems a sure sign of a passive character and indifferent fathering, then one should simply change the perspective from that of judging parental performance to that of assessing marital loyalty and support. From that perspective, one sees that Mr. Fletcher is sensitive to his wife's need for dominion over the children as her pathway to identity and to containment of her anxieties about men. Now one may label him as perceptive and loyal. It simply requires a change of context and an entering into the transactional field from a new perspective. One changes viewpoint, as though watching Mr. Fletcher were like looking at a single bit of colored glass in a kaleidoscopic pattern. In the total family context, this colored bit fits imperfectly and is lodged on the edge of some larger, multicolored design that seems barely to include him and certainly not to need him. If the kaleidoscope is turned slightly, then the bit that is Mr. Fletcher swiftly falls into the center of a new pattern, one which is equally interesting in its color and complexity, but which now requires his centrality to give coherence to the total design. In turning the kaleidoscope, one has altered the context of perception and has found a different meaning for Mr. Fletcher's quietness. One has reframed his behavior and has done so in a positive way.

Many good psychotherapies do just this, though it may be called by other names. Certainly, psychoanalysis, if it is to be helpful at all, offers analysands an increasingly complex picture of their particular behaviors, thereby offering them the chance to reframe their behaviors in more positive ways. It is axiomatic that when one introduces complexity—whether into a perception of another's experience or the understanding of one's own—then one creates a new context allowing a more positive verdict on life.

A NOTE ON CONTEXTUAL COMPLEXITY

A brief elaboration on the merits of contextual complexity may be helpful at this point. In common parlance, complexity, when applied to psychological matters, often connotes a greater confusion of entangled perspectives than is really necessary to understand something. Therapists are said to make matters unnecessarily complex when more simple formulations would do just as well. Hence, to call for complexity in viewing the context of symptomatic behavior does not seem, initially, of any great benefit to either client or therapist. Complexity is equated with muddiness; it is the opposite of clear simplicity.

In systems theory, however, the meaning of complexity is quite different. From a systems viewpoint, any particular behavior has more power and fewer meanings (including some possibly positive meanings) the more simple its contextual surrounding is. Conversely, the more complex the surrounding, the greater is the number of meanings that may be assigned to a particular behavior, and the less susceptible the total context is to being influenced by that single behavioral event. Consider the diagram presented in Figure 7-1, which shows that in moving from context 1 to context 3, the power of the "dot" to organize its context becomes less, while its possible meanings multiply. Where the context is primitively organized, as in the first instance, any given behavior is assigned a simple meaning and has considerable power to affect the overall functioning of the larger context. This condition is associated with rigid systems behavior, moralistic and inflexible judgments of the behavior involved, and little opportunity for fresh views of what is causing the problem. As one moves to a more evolved organization of the context, i.e., where complexity of meaning is introduced, then the determining power of the dot is less, and there is greater flexibility in the overall system, as well as a greater opportunity for new and more positive views of any given behavior. From the systems viewpoint, complexity in the interpersonal context is a necessary precondition for the positive reframing of symptomatic behaviors.

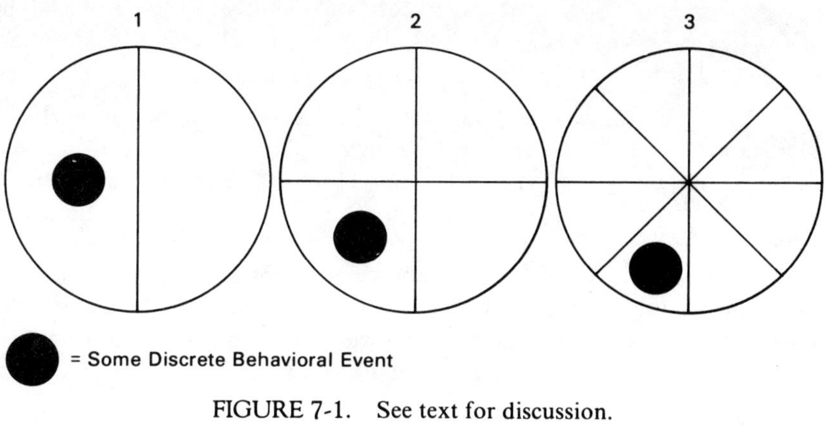

FIGURE 7-1. See text for discussion.

Reframing is good psychotherapy and is not special to the structural approach as such, although Minuchin, who has focused some attention on the need to create new realities and new belief systems for troubled families (Minuchin & Fishman, 1981), might in fact argue that positive reframing is precisely what good structural family therapists do, since their job is to create new contexts for behavior. New contexts develop when, via positive reframing, complexity is introduced into the cognitive schemes of individual family members. But the introduction of complexity is common to most effective psychotherapies. Therefore, one can argue either that something "structural" is common to all psychotherapies (probably true) or that this particular feature of structural family therapy occurs simply because it is *a* psychotherapy, one invariant aspect of which is the use of positive relabeling. The latter seems the best argument, although one could add that there may be something distinctively "structural" about the examples of positive reframing reported here—namely, that the reframing is used to prepare a part of the system that previously was not much used as an information pathway and to arrange for that part to become an active conveyor of new viewpoints. Reframing, in this way, becomes restructuring.

Telling, teaching, explaining, and interpreting are all ways of trying to change families by enlisting them as observers of their own transaction experiences. Through these varieties of bringing consciousness to others, the therapist tries to enrich the contextual meaning of a particular symptomatic behavior, thereby rendering that behavior more susceptible to change. Therapists, however, are not the only ones who seek new explanations for behavior and change; families do also, and often in ways that assault the sanctity of therapeutic explanation. Everyone has a cautionary tale about the helpfulness of explanation in creating change. Here is one such story.

Clyde and the Virgin

Clyde, age 10, was the youngest of four children in a poor working-class family. The parents were undereducated, hard working, and devoted to their family. Clyde was the pride of the family. He was gifted at school, successful with his peers, and helpful around the house. One day, however, Clyde decided not to go to school. He became school-phobic and was as successful at that as he had been elsewhere in his life. After a month of entreaties, punishments, and consultations with the family doctor, the parents brought Clyde to treatment. He was a charming boy, neatly dressed and wearing a tie. He was adept at light conversation, and his usual cheerfulness was marred only by his adamant refusal to go to school. His parents had tried everything, but Clyde was triumphant. If, for example, they physically threw him out of the house, he would break in the door with ferocious strength and then spend the remainder of the day repairing it, using his father's tool kit with great skill. The mother and father were proud of his repair work, but puzzled about his "sickness."

The therapist made several usual moves. The mother was failing to get up in the mornings and was instead staying in bed, "going through the change" with great turmoil, which included suffering many "hot flashes." In fact, she enjoyed Clyde's company during the day. After the early morning struggle, which took place after the father had left for work, the mother and Clyde would settle in to watch the morning soap operas, do a bit of cooking together, and generally enjoy each other. The father was not aware of this, since neither his wife nor Clyde was innocent enough to tell. The therapist made a successful alliance with the father, met with the marital couple to increase the father's understanding of how his wife was feeling at this particular time in her life, and finally, got the wife to begin leaving home each morning to visit with friends down the block. The father was helped to understand that Clyde was worried his mother might be sick (after all, she stayed in bed a good deal and complained even more) and that a father's firm hand would be more than welcome. So the father arranged to go to work late for several mornings while his wife got up, dressed, and left the house to spend the morning with friends. Clyde soon returned to school, where the father and the therapist had already met with the teacher to secure his support for Clyde's return. The parents were pleased, and Clyde's classmates were glad to have him back.

Three months later, the therapist called to do a follow-up. Since Clyde was still in school and the mother still on her feet, the family members agreed to come to the clinic for a single interview, although they had already forgotten the therapist's name. During the interview, the therapist asked the parents about their understanding of Clyde's recovery. The mother offered the following: During the mornings that she had been required to leave the house, letting her husband attend to Clyde, she had in fact gone to early Mass, where she lit candles to the Virgin and prayed for Clyde's recovery. Having made this alliance with the Virgin instead of with her neighbors, as she had promised the therapist, the mother felt guilty and finally confessed to her husband. The husband felt sympathetic toward her and agreed that they should keep this a secret from the therapist who, after all, seemed well intentioned and had many ideas about why Clyde stayed at home. At any rate, they were grateful for divine intervention and for Clyde's miraculous cure; and they felt that the therapy had at least done no harm.

SUMMARY

This chapter, and the one preceding it, reviewed those intervention strategies classically associated with structural family therapy. They are (1) crisis induction, (2) treatment staging, (3) the analysis of structure over content, (4) intervention into hierarchies and sequences, (5) task assignments, and (6) the use of explanation and description. The application of these techniques summarizes the structural approach. There is a consistent emphasis on the analysis of structure and on the interruption of behavioral sequences that make up unhappy alliances and troubled hierarchies. Interventions are applied at the interface between two subsystems that are contiguous and that form the context within which individual symptoms occur. The interventions all require considerable therapist activity and assume a capacity to recast immense amounts of data into a structural map and structural hypothesis about the family problem. But "classic moves" are not always enough, and therapy sometimes falters. What is one to do when the good moves are gone?

Chapter 8

In the Middle and Beyond

From the perspective of many students, family therapy often seems an exercise in brilliant openings and happy outcomes with little in between worth mentioning. Is there, one wonders, life after the initial interview? There is—and it is a great midland of effort and failure, of progress and resistance to progress. It is a land of mucky middles where the momentum of the initial phase is often lost, replaced by the unromantic trudge of a therapist and a family who struggle toward change. Troubles and resistances are inevitable, but they are also instructive. Families without lively resistance may in fact be living systems without much life left in them. In a truly lively family, uneven progress and periodic retrenchment are virtual certainties. This chapter traces the family therapy experiences of the Fletcher family as they unfold after the initial interview. Periodic asides highlight instances of resistance and special questions common to most family therapy cases. This chapter suggests how to address these resistances and how to recover from a failed intervention. To begin, a word about resistance in systems seems in order.

RESISTANCE IN SYSTEMS

Except for families who enter treatment in an acute crisis, most troubled families have a faint air of chronicity about their living arrangements. The therapist, as Minuchin and Fishman (1981, p.20) have noted, encounters these powerful and controlling stabilizing mechanisms much more readily than he or she encounters the family's capacity for change. Moreover, this powerful stability appears in the worst of systemic routines, even where the cost to certain individuals is extraordinarily high. A general rule is that the higher the cost the more rigid the system. In short, to discover a family group operating at a considerable expense to its members should not encourage the therapist to believe that this group is ready to change. For that matter, all systems, from the most rigid to the least, are essentially conservative and must undergo persistent environmental persuasions before altering the routines of a lifetime. It is naturally the intention of the therapist to create, with the family as partner, just such a persuasive environment. This therapeutic endeavor can be more happily pursued when the therapist accepts that any system has normal limits that regulate the rate at which and extent to which change may occur. In this way, "resistance" is not pathological, but only another version of a system's propensity to regulate itself. These limits to growth are a kind of regulatory setting that persists until the family moves to a different level of systemic organization. Resistance, as a formal term, refers to (1) the temporal and energetic inertia of a system to alter the behavioral strategies that (2) serve to maintain a stasis that proves tolerable enough (3) between those parts of the system that are structurally related to the particular behavioral process labeled as symptomatic.

Whether this process of change is sudden, involving a kind of "evolutionary leap," as Hoffman (1980) and Dell (1982) have suggested, or something more continuous and gradual is a matter beyond the present inquiry. The nature and process of change is enormously complex, but the phenomenal reality of resistance to it is well known to any clinician.

In addition to the resistance to change that is healthily inherent in all systems, there is the resistance of each component part to changes in adjacent parts of the whole. When interventions pose greater threats than advantages to an individual's subsystem membership, greater resistance to change will exist. This is a potential problem since each family member belongs to several subsystems. A husband and wife are both marital partners and parents. Children are members of their sibling group, but are also children of their parents. All have simultaneous membership in their total family unit and in the surrounding culture. When an intervention seems stuck and change resisted, it may be, for example, that the threats to an adult's position as a marital partner greatly outweigh the benefits to his or her position as a parent. Resistance to the intervention will be correspondingly high. If being allowed a strategy for better parenting inadvertently creates a problem in the marital system, then the therapist may find a good intervention mysteriously blocked. Since each person occupies some interface ground between adjacent subsystems, interventions requiring new behavior in the first system inevitably have consequences for behavior in the second system. As an example, consider the man who is not getting along with his wife, a woman his family warned him against marrying because she was from another ethnic and class background. If he follows the therapist's interventions into the marriage and begins to get along better with his wife, he is making yet another betrayal of his extended family, which has instructed him *not* to get along with her. The husband must weigh the relative advantages to his membership in each subsystem before he changes his behavior. In addition, it would not be surprising to find a person poised at that interface to be symptomatic.

CHANGING THE FLETCHERS

The work of therapy in the middle phases, the issues of change and resistance, are clearly present in the treatment of the Fletcher family. At the end of the initial interviewing phase, the therapist summarized his impressions with a diagnostic map (see Fig. 4-9, p. 75) and a written note (Chapter 4). That note was the therapist's structural hypothesis and stated the following: Within the context of a deep schism dividing men from women, Irving's symptoms reflect his absence of core membership in a firmly identified male subgroup, complete with the male models so needed in adolescence, and his unwitting role in helping his mother reaffirm both the tight boundaries of the women's group and her place within it. Without the reinforcement of these symptomatic behaviors, Judy might be freed to move away from her mother and eventually away from home, as her older sisters have done. This would leave the mother more available to possible connections with her husband. Or, stated from the husband's position, if he were more forcefully to initiate behaviors that would help his children differentiate from the larger family unit by joining their appropriate subsystems, he would be positioned to have more contact with his wife. The son's symptoms and the family response to them form behavioral sequences that prevent this from happening.

With this summary in mind, the therapist could imagine several stages in the treatment process, beginning with an effort to get Mr. Fletcher more involved with his sons. While these initial plans will be modified by the evolving realities of the therapeutic process, beginning with a clear treatment proposal establishes a sense of seriousness and hope in both the family and the therapist. The plan envisioned by the therapist, though not shared with the family beyond a discussion of the first stage, is presented in Table 8-1.

Stage 1: Father and Sons

At the end of the initial interview, the therapist decided, on the basis of his initial diagnostic map (Fig. 4-9), that the first stage of treatment should involve Mr. Fletcher and his sons, with the wife and daughters carefully

Table 8-1
THERAPIST'S PLAN FOR TREATMENT OF THE FLETCHER FAMILY

Stage	Subsystem	Goals
1	Father and sons	To empower the peripheral father, to develop a men's subsystem with an articulated boundary, and to help Irving feel located within that group, and thereby able to assume an identity with men—Bob and his father—who were effective in the outer world, as Irving was not.
2	All children	To help the siblings see themselves as distinct from the parents and as having common issues among themselves; to help them appreciate differences between those siblings still living at home and those living outside the home.
3	Entire family	To test the viability of new subsystem boundaries, to assess the status of Irving's symptoms, and to intervene directly into the family routines built around them.
4	Parents alone	To assess and address issues that have arisen between the parents and to indicate the right of parents to be separate from the children as a distinct subunit.
5	Parents and children living at home	To emphasize the integrity of *this* family, composed of those children still at home plus the parents, and the need to address the life-cycle needs of this group.

assigned a secondary role. He therefore, with the children present, issued such an invitation to the father. It was carefully phrased to take note of Mrs. Fletcher's need for some relief from her struggle with Irving, and it assumed a benevolent wish on her husband's part to "help out the whole family." The focus on the men was also based on the therapist's need to know more about them, since they would be primarily responsible for helping Irving, a suggestion to which no one responded with any interest. Still, both parents and Irving agreed to this invitation, and the father planned to call his older son, Bob. At the next meeting, a week later, Mr. Fletcher and Bob arrived for the interview. Irving, however, stayed at home.

When Staging Fails

To have an opening move fail may signal a basic flaw in the treatment planning, though such a flaw is rarely apparent until the therapist makes a detailed inquiry. There are many ways to reach a restructuring goal, and hence other staging strategies may be required. If interventions into one subsystem are met only with resistance, the therapist should rapidly consider other alternative groupings.

What should *not* be considered is any further assessment of the individual symptom bearer, always a temptation at this juncture. Just as the family has organized itself to ignore larger flaws and focus instead on one person, so too will it try to organize the therapist into a similar position. The therapist who is inducted here will forget about a family approach and decide that some additional evaluation of the troubled individual is called for, perhaps including some diagnostic testing. The family will be without resistance to this suggestion and will rapidly produce the patient. Thus warned, the savvy therapist simply assesses why the staging did not work and gives up the initial plan only with thoughtful reluctance; otherwise, the therapist should keep the plan and work through the resistances to it. One of the dangers of the family approach is also its blessing—namely, that therapists have access to a number of different family groupings, all of which may offer different approaches to solving the problem. This very diversity, however, can also lead the therapist to abandon too easily the initial staging plan, flitting from one family group to another until all credibility and planning is lost. Hence, as with all failed tasks, the therapist's first response is to make a detailed inquiry into the circumstances of failure.

In the case of the Fletchers, the therapist assumed there would be some resistance to this staging move, since it would make the father more central and the mother less so. Whether the father's centrality was the source of resistance would not be clear until an inquiry was made. As the therapist listened to Mr. Fletcher's account of what happened, it became clear that Mr. Fletcher felt ill prepared to deal with an "emotional son" like Irving. Using frequent references to Bob, who sat by comfortably and without comment, Mr. Fletcher described his feeling that Irving was different from himself and Bob. He and Bob simply left their homes early, found good jobs, and felt firmly identified with their place in the world of work. It appeared that Bob had conformed nicely to this developmental script, entering the Army shortly after his graduation from high school and then, later, into a low-level computer programming field where he now held steady employment. With Bob, Mr. Fletcher was spared any introspective concern about his abilities as a father. Irving's behavior, on the other hand, embarrassed him and, he hinted, exposed him to considerable criticism from his wife. Thus, when the day arrived for the interview, Mr. Fletcher found himself feeling irritable, on edge, and angry at Irving—quite the opposite of what the therapist hoped. During breakfast, Irving became involved in a minor fight with Judy, and Mr. Fletcher found himself getting very angry and threatening to "tell the therapist" and to get him to "put Irving away." Irving bolted from the room, saying he was not going to the meeting. The father made no protest; Irving did not appear at the session.

Mr. Fletcher seemed disturbed and even guilty about these events. He hinted at other issues in his life that in the past had made him less than a good father, but seemed understandably reluctant to discuss them in front of Bob. The therapist listened in a sympathetic way and tried to explore how the father and brother might work together to get Irving to come in the following week. There was, however, little energy between Mr. Fletcher and Bob, and there was no particular history that Bob shared with Irving, though he did not seem antagonistic toward him. There simply were no developed dyadic alliances among the male members of the family. Given this and the father's apparent willingness to say more about himself, the therapist suggested that he and Mr. Fletcher alone get together to discuss further how to deal with this very difficult situation. The intention was to accept a slowing-down of the staging process (recognizing that the breakfast-table episode had already introduced a regulatory rhythm that could not be easily challenged) and to allow the father to enter into some alliance with the therapist, a move that would itself be a model for the alliance building between men that was needed in this family. With this kind of reframing and rehearsal, the first stage of treatment could remain as the transacting of business between father and sons. Offering some individual time to Mr. Fletcher endorsed his membership in the parenting hierarchy (presently a subgroup principally occupied by Mrs. Fletcher and Judy). In this family, it would have been a mistake to offer the individual consultations to the mother, since she, and not the father, was the parent who customarily made alliances outside the family. For her to meet with the therapist, leaving her husband once more on the periphery, would simply have continued a dysfunctional family pattern.

Meeting With Individuals

This strategy for dealing with resistance to an initial staging move demonstrates how family therapists may meet with single individuals in order to pursue wider structural goals. Meetings to rehearse new behaviors and to gain a sympathetic understanding of one person's life story are not contraindicated by the structural approach. On the contrary, when key individuals in the system need preparation time and when contact with them does not perpetuate a structural flaw in the family, therapists may arrange for such meetings. These meetings should be time limited and primarily in the service of helping that individual move into a restructured position within the larger family, especially in the immediate weeks ahead as the therapy progresses.

The therapist and Mr. Fletcher met twice. The therapist, with a sense of kindly regard, reviewed Mr. Fletcher's life story, particularly those details connected with his parenting, which included some information about his own father. To minimize Mrs. Fletcher's worry that nothing was being done during this time about the real problem, Irving, the therapist suggested to Mr. Fletcher that he advise his wife that he was preparing to "speak with Irving" and that she should practice not responding to him, but instead let Judy handle her own fights.

Throughout these individual meetings, the therapist encouraged Mr. Fletcher to urge Irving to bring him all his complaints about his mother and sisters. While Irving was not in any way required to alter his actual pattern of fights (for Irving had much to defend), he was expected to let his father know a lot about his problems. The therapist acknowledged to Mr. Fletcher that it would be hard to hear from his "emotional son," but added that he had the backing of the therapist and that his wife would surely appreciate Mr. Fletcher's efforts. Nothing was to change except the procedure of reporting. There were to be no punishments and no requests that Irving and Judy avoid each other. These arrangements were carefully rehearsed with the father and, during one week, were confirmed by a short phone call from him to the therapist. Mr. Fletcher announced this change in reporting to his wife and Judy as well as to Irving. He carried out his end of it quite well, as did Irving, who in fact succeeded in keeping the incidence of his misbehavior fairly high. This continuing trouble seemed to indicate that while the bonding with the father was important, Irving was still caught in routines that were part of larger family issues.

During the two weeks following his individual contacts with the therapist, Mr. Fletcher and both sons arrived for the meetings. With help, they discussed what it had been like for the sons to grow up in the family, why the two brothers were not more close, and why the men never seemed to do much together. During these conversations, Bob and his father sat in separate chairs on one side of the room, near the door, while the therapist and Irving found themselves grouped together on the opposite side. The seating may have been inadvertent, but it dramatized the point that even when the men were together, Irving was left out. In the middle of the second meeting, as Irving began his usual litany of charges, especially the charge that his father never took his side in the fights with the mother or with Judy, there occurred the following exchange:

Irving: (To the father) You never say a thing, no matter whay *they* do. You never believe me!

Father: I don't really know who's right. Your mother gets really upset with you, so. . . .

Irving: (Angrily) There it is. There you are, taking her side again. Not mine.

Therapist: (To Irving) Even now, I imagine you feel your father could never be on your side. Look where he is sitting—so far away there with Bob. You are left out even here in this room. Maybe if you pulled your chair closer to him, kind of got into their circle, why then this business of "sides" might not be so big. Try moving over there a bit.

Irving: (Very upset and angry) To hell with that. He'll never do anything. I won't give him nothing. To hell with him . . . he just hates me.

The group was stunned by this outburst, and the therapist worried that Irving was losing control. The atmosphere was tense, but the therapist decided to press on in a different way, still on the track of an alliance between Irving and his father.

Therapist: (To Irving) Well, look, just hold it a bit. Just be cool. That was wrong of me . . . I don't get it yet, but I know, in spite of how angry you are, that you hate being left out from them. So here's what. Don't move at all, stay sitting right there. O.K. But now do this: just relax and stay right there, but I want you to *imagine* you and your father sitting together. Just get a mental picture of the two of you being together while you talk.

Irving: (Beginning to cry softly) I hate this. I don't want this fight with you. I don't want this. . . .

Father: (Shifting uncomfortably in his seat and leaning forward) Don't get so upset. Let's just forget this stuff. I know you didn't mean all that (said kindly).

Therapist: (To the father) That's good, you're reaching a bit to let him know, you know, that you can really see his side of things. That will help a lot.

Father: I really can, actually, and, Irv, I really know it's not all you. Don't get so upset now. (The father is awkward with the feelings.)

Irving: I'm all right now. Forget it. It's all right. Let's go on.

The tone in the room shifted from anger to sadness, and the tension was gone.

Imagery and Structure

Irving's resistance to an actual alteration of physical distance between himself and his father was understandable. It was an error for the therapist to ask Irving to contact his peripheral father, since the father's distancing was part of what Irving was already angry about. The instruction to make yet another effort enraged him. On the other hand, Irving certainly had some positive feelings toward his father, and these needed to be elicited if any alliance was to develop between the two of them. At this point, the therapist continued the intervention, but he switched from a behavioral manipulation (changing chairs) to the elicitation of internal imagery in the individual. He gave the son permission *not to move in reality,* but to do so only *in imagination.* Freed of the negative emotions engendered by the prospect of making a move to the distant father, the son could sit quietly while briefly overcome by his more positive yearnings to be with his father. His crying prompted a care-giving response from his father, who made an actual behavioral gesture when he leaned forward in his chair, as though to reach out to Irving. He consoled him with his voice, even while telling him to suppress the emotions. The therapist, aware that this arrangement—namely, one where the *father* moved toward the son—was correct, supported Mr. Fletcher, praising him for seeing his son's side of the problem. The emotional tone shifted from tense anger to calm sadness.

This example demonstrates how inner psychological events can be used to achieve changes in interpersonal structure. When the Fletcher's therapist shifted from behavior to the *imagined* rehearsal for behavior (a mental picture of sitting with the father), the son was freed to experience a new emotion, and an opportunity arose for the father to respond in a different way. In general, structural therapy can use individual internal events in the service of interpersonal goals. By focusing on an internal, imagined event, the Fletcher men were able to experience a new emotion and then to behave differently toward each other. A shift in the emotional field facilitated a shift in behavioral transactions. In transactions like this one, structural therapy is a cybernetic process; behavior (sometimes imagined behavior) engenders new emotions, and these, in turn, allow new behaviors. (See also the earlier remarks on a general plan for structural change, Chapter 2.)

Stage 2: The Fletcher Children

The therapist had several options at this point. Had there been more time, he might have held some parallel meetings with Mrs. Fletcher and her daughters, meetings intended to establish a more differentiated subgroup. If the issue with the men was their lack of cohesiveness, and hence some fragmentation of their individual identities as men, then the reverse problem was true with the women, who were too tightly bound with each other, a tradition beginning with Mrs. Fletcher's overinvolvement with her own mother. While the men needed cohesion and unity, the women needed differentiation and diversity.

The therapist decided to address these issues by meeting directly with all the children in order to establish their differences from the parents. In a telephone call to Mrs. Fletcher, the therapist repeated what he had said to Mr. Fletcher during their last meeting—that it was natural in late adolescence for the children to get together and find common interests. The parents should trust the children to undertake this task fairly. He also suggested to Mrs. Fletcher that in the next week, during the evening time when he was meeting with the children, she and her husband should go out to dinner in order to remind each other that they had been good parents. This was a suggestion that made no obvious sense and yet seemed harmless enough since it said nothing specifically about their getting together as marital partners. They agreed to this, and a meeting was scheduled with the children.

There were several intentions here. First, it was an opportunity to see Irving in yet another context. Previously, he had been seen with his brother and father and, before that, with the entire family. Now he could be seen with no parent present. Throughout the interview, he was more reasonable and much less volatile than in previous meetings; his encounters with Judy were surprisingly soft, even friendly. They joked on occasion and teased each other pleasantly. The single angry moment for Irving came when his older sisters, Mary and Eileen, were discussing their growing up at home. When the therapist asked about their father, they responded coolly and briefly, assuming a critical attitude toward him. Irving responded angrily, claiming they were "stuck up" and "full of it" and "always on Mother's side." This suggested an additional burden expressed through his symptoms—that of representing the father and of being the father's proxy in a family fight that had gone on for some years.

This meeting was also an opportunity to promote a clearer boundary between the older children and the parents. If successful, it would (1) be another way of helping Judy and Irving reduce their overinvolvement with the mother and (2) indirectly leave the parents to wander around in the same social plane, perhaps to link up with each other more than had been the case so far. Actually, this boundary making was not difficult, for aside from the daughters' nearly unanimous support of their mother, they all felt basic permission to get on with their lives. The older sisters felt Judy should leave home during the coming year, but they had no opinion about Irving. During this meeting, the therapist attempted to promote as much affiliation between the two brothers as existed among the sisters. He met with only modest success. Throughout the interview, the therapist persisted in defining the brothers as a unit, reminding them of their joint meetings with the father and of the things they had shared together, without becoming specific about content. Bob was offered the role of a helpful big brother, and the therapist described sympathetically how all three men in the family were somehow isolated, noting that male isolation was more a cultural problem than a problem peculiar to their particular family.

The response to this comment about isolation was unexpected, for Janice, age 10, who had been generally neglected by everyone, began to cry. She said that of all the children, she was the one who had no friends in the family except her mother. Indeed, she was too young to be naturally included in the older girls' group, and it was equally difficult to place her with the boys. She showed surprising sympathy for Irving and great energy in pursuing her own complaints. The therapist noted that just as Bob needed to be an "older brother" to Irving, especially in showing Irving how to make it in the world, Judy needed to be a good "older sister" to Janice and to find ways to make her feel more accepted. Mary and Eileen had already been defined as "older sisters" to Judy and as her guides out of the home. In this way, the sibling group was differentiated into hierarchies of older and younger and of those making it in the world and those preparing to do so. Their energies and allegiances were directed toward each other and the outside world, leaving them less available to their parents, who would have to redefine the meaning of their unit once all the children except Janice were gone.

Tracking and Persistence

In many of these meetings, the therapist was required to persist in tracking the divergent expressions of a main theme. Persistence is a good antidote to certain resistances, especially those that can be labeled more as habit than as pathological necessity. In the Fletchers, for example, it had become a habit to consider the men as socially isolated within the family unit; Irving tried to break that habit by complaining (calling for help) about his placement in these routines. Therapists in general, when convinced of the utility of an announced theme, must keep track of its many manifestations and not hesitate persistently to promote new behavioral routines that can alter the major theme. As Minuchin and Fishman have noted, "Systems have an inertia that resists change, and repetition is required for repatterning to occur. Therapy is a matter of repetition . . ."(1981, p.123). This persistence is useful, whether attending to the large themes of family life or to the small details of who sits where or who always speaks first as opposed to who always speaks last. When alterations in these patterns are framed as useful and of demonstrated value, there is nothing embarrassing about persistently helping people to continue the changes.

In the Fletcher case, such persistence was apparent when, for example, the therapist constantly supported the father's usefulness as a more central parent or, as discussed below, always arranged for Irving to sit with his father and brother rather than to occupy his usual place among the women. At other points, he was similarly persistent in not allowing the mother to speak for Judy; he correctly assumed that if Judy were allowed time to finish full statements of her sentiments, a substantial conflict would arise between her and her mother, and that this crisis would be necessary to continue the process of change. Too frequently, therapists develop a useful intervention, drop it into the family pool, and then fail to observe its ripple. They need to track its effect, both immediate and delayed, as well as to persist in the intervention when it clearly brings about a more healthy context for family business.

Stage 3: The Whole Family

Meeting with the entire Fletcher family was critical and involved a number of intentions: (1) to assess any positive effects of the subunit definitions that the therapist had been promoting; (2) to assess, through report and observation, the status of Irving's symptoms; (3) to allow the father to take more of a central role than he did in the initial interview; (4) to allow parental differences to surface, perhaps as a consequence of the father's possible assumption of this more central role; and finally (5) to locate and disrupt, during the interview, the dysfunctional sequences diagnosed in the initial interview.

In the opening minutes of this interview, there was an opportunity to define subunit boundaries by using a standard intervention around seating patterns. The family entered and arranged themselves in a manner similar to that of the initial meeting. Irving was sitting between Judy and Eileen, far removed from his father, who sat with the older son, across the room and near the door. Before any substantive conversation could begin, the therapist successfully rearranged the seating. He invited Irving to leave his place among the sisters and, trading places with Janice, to move over next to his father and Bob. Looking directly at Irving, the therapist said, "This is not where you were sitting when we talked last, with all your sisters, I mean. I think it's easier to keep it all straight when you and your father are closer to the action. So trade with Janice here, and then . . . it will be a better place." This comment was a mixture of accurate description and optimistic suggestion, and coming so early in the interview, before people were settled in, it easily succeeded. It is not always so easy, however.

Changing Seats: Resistance in Place

Parodies of structural family therapy are easy and entertaining, beginning with spoofs of the therapist who creates a game of musical chairs and who constantly moves people from place to place. The musical track consists of the therapist making clever "reframing" remarks that justify why people are switching chairs to sit with other people they obviously don't like. Or the therapist is depicted as blocking a child from intruding into the "marital space" by extending an arm between the child and parents, each family unit looking longingly at the other like neighborly countries separated by a fascist wall. Actually, seat changing and the physical signals indicating that certain family members should now be quiet are frequently used in an effort to help people visualize a rearrangement of family structure and to *feel* what it would be like to live in that new space. Children who are terribly caught up in their parents' issues will, for example, frequently report their relief that the therapist moved them from the immediate interview circle, perhaps to a seat just outside the group, and then took their place in mediating the parents' fight. Conversely, the longing to be closer, to be more in alliance with someone, is often facilitated by an experimental manipulation of seating.

For structuralists, the medium is often the message; what people are saying is less important than arranging a structure syntonic with the message. If, for example, the parents agree to talk together, but continue to have their three children arrayed between them, it is hard to know how serious the parents' effort to talk will be. In addition, when a therapist instructs two people to talk together, no one need take that instruction seriously unless there is a simultaneous arrangement of the interview and seating space so that the people really are positioned to talk. (Alterations in seating and spatial distance must, of course, be consistent with the cultural and ethnic values of any particular client.) Forms of staging, subgrouping, and actual dividing of the interview into a time for parents and children together followed by a time for the spouses alone are all instructions about seating and, often, instructions about speaking that are designed to give the family a visual and emotional opportunity to adapt to new structures. In part, this is the intent of family sculpture, though that has never become an important technique of structural therapy, since sculpture has traditionally placed so much emphasis on internal feeling states.

This very ordinary, everyday technique, however, produces some of the worst moments in a therapist's life. The technique itself is generally presented in this way:

Therapist: (Speaking to the parents) It would be great if you could continue this, about how to raise the kids and so on. But how about changing seats with them, so they are not in the middle, so you are actually together.

Therapists may then gesture, assume an expectant look, or with real presence of mind, actually get up from their own chair, thereby providing a clear example of what is expected. Here are some of the responses that quickly will lower therapists back to ground level:

Father: This is just fine, we always sit like this because we want the children to feel included. (The implication is that the therapist has tried to impose an unwelcome and undemocratic value system on the family.)

OR

Mother: What's wrong with where I am? There's too much going on here . . . I can't see what you want from us. (The mother personalizes the request and feels criticized.)

OR

Father: (To the therapist) Don't be silly! Now where were we? (As Graham Greene noted in *Our Man in Havana,* some people expect to be tortured, others do not. Some expect displacement, others know exactly where they wish to sit.)

Finally, other resistances may be total silence from the family or some obvious signs of discomfort from the children, especially the index child, who is usually most sensitive to alterations in the parental dyad. Therapists, of course, feel quite compromised and powerless, returning foolishly to their seat.

The recovery from this embarrassment may take two forms, both designed to help the therapist learn more about the family. The first is a more provocative pronouncement, made to the entire family:

Therapist: I guess mom and dad are not quite ready to be so much in the same boat after all.

OR

I guess the kids are not quite ready to let you two get together.

These remarks presume that the therapist has additional information that makes them more than just provocative; without such information, the hole only gets deeper. A safer recovery rests on a simple description of the family's response to the therapist's request:

Therapist: I've just stubbed my toe on one of your family rules, some rule about where the kids can be when the parents are having grownup talk. Who can tell me what I missed and just what happened here?

Whatever the recovery technique, a persistent inquiry into the rules that make up resistance to seating changes can reveal to the therapist new and valuable information about family structure.

In the Fletchers' case, the seating change evoked a mild flurry of activity on the part of the mother and Janice, who giggled as she switched her seat and moved closer to her sisters and mother. The meeting began with a review of the weeks during which some members of the family had not seen the therapist, but soon settled into what promised to be a favorite scapegoating routine. According to the mother, Irving's behavior had not changed much; according to the father, it was reported to be better. This difference of opinion would soon be useful. The real event of note in this interview came midway through, as criticism of Irving mounted. It was a familiar sequence involving the mother, Judy, and Irving, a sequence the therapist now tried to stop by using Mrs. Fletcher as the leading edge of change.

The therapist and the mother were discussing how well most of her children had turned out and how she was puzzled by Irving.

Therapist: So, like with Eileen and Mary, it's a good job, and now I know you're proud with Judy and Janice. Good kids. (He looks at them.) Your mother feels you are a kind of testament to her being at home all these years.

Mother: Oh no. They are fine. I tried, but they have been wonderful. Most of the time. (Laughs.)

Therapist: So I kind of wonder when they all leave, well, say, when Judy leaves, which she could do next year. Just what you will do for a living. Looks like early retirement.

Mother: Ah, no. Judy has lots of time, especially. . . .

Judy: To enter legal work, I really would need to start work *and* get into school. (She was planning on becoming a legal secretary.)

Mother: Right. So with money and all, I see it that you will need all the support we can give. Here at home.

Judy: Yeah, but I also could live away. Share an apartment or something.

Mother: Yeah (laughs), . . . that's kind of unrealistic. I think, when you figure it all out, that being here for a while makes good sense. (There is now an air of impending sharpness between the mother and Judy.)

Irving: (To the mother) How do you know everything all the time? You don't know nothing.

Mother: I know you won't go any place unless you straighten up.

Judy: (To Irving) Just shut up . . . bug off, and. . . .

Irving: (Angrily) I've got a right to speak when I want and. . . .

Therapist: (Interrupting Irving and looking at the father) I think you better step in here. Because this happens a lot. Judy and her mother have this problem about discussing her leaving home, and then Irv tries to help out by sort of distracting everything onto himself. Then your wife and Judy are pals again, until the next time. Why don't you help Irv hold it down, tell him not to worry about them so much. Your wife and daughter can work this out. Can you do that?

Father: (He looks at the therapist, but makes no response.)

Therapist: (To Mrs. Fletcher and Judy) You have a real difference here, so go ahead. You don't need Irving to protect you from having real differences.

Irving: (To the therapist) You got it all wrong. They will never settle that. They. . . .

Therapist: (Interrupting Irving; to the father) This is the point right here. See? Can you get your son to cool it for a while? So they can talk.

Father: O.K., son. Try it, try it just for now. (Said quietly, but with some clear intention that Irving should obey.)

Therapist: Good. Now you two go on.

Interrupting Sequences

Resistance to sequence interruption is greatest with dealing with broad macroscopic events. It is often difficult for the therapist to get the correct picture at first, since so much may depend on report rather than direct observation. Moreover, the labeling of people's behavior as competent or incompetent, as Haley (1976) has done, is delicate, to say the least, and it is difficult to agree on the labels used. On the other hand, description of and intervention into the isomorphic microsequences, as they occur in the interview room, are more successful. Such interventions are the preferred way to alter sequences and to deal with resistance to changes in the larger sequences. The description can take place in a routine manner, the behavioral experience is often quite apparent once it is mentioned, and the family will tend to alter its behavior rather than struggle with the therapist. Once family members have some practice in accepting and altering these miniaturized analogs of the larger sequences, which may be spread over many hours or days, they can be encouraged to address the experiential sequences that occur at home.

In the example above, a crucial exchange (without doubt a parallel to the events at home) was addressed and altered. The sequence was a familiar one for the Fletchers. Judy's rehearsals to leave home seemed threatening to her mother who, in her efforts to discourage her daughter, was indirectly helped by Irving, who drew Judy into a fight. As the mother defended Judy, she and her daughter again ended up in a tight dyad in which legitimate conflict could not surface. The therapist tried to accomplish several things with his comment about this small exchange. He labeled the mother and Judy as having a problem, a statement that previously had never been made openly. He positively labeled Irving as trying to help them both out. The major structural move was to try and involve the father in the effective regulation of the sequence by siding with his son *and* assuming the authority to pronounce that his "wife and daughter can work this out." This put the father back inside the family in an effective place in the presenting hierarchy. Although his initial response was not forceful, the father clearly had the idea and showed some determination to proceed with it. Even if the father's initial response was not as energetic as one would wish, one may assume that this sequence, in varied forms, will repeat itself and that the therapist will repeatedly make the *same* intervention. Persistence in this matter was an important key to helping the family label and alter these sequences. Note that in this example of the Fletcher family, as in most cases, a sequence was successfully interrupted when cross-generational misalliances were challenged and when the symptomatic person's behavior was positively redefined as inevitable, given the current structural arrangement. Change here came about when the father replaced Irving as the mother's ally, supporting her right to deal competently with her daughter and freeing his son from distracting his mother through his symptomatic angers.

Mrs. Fletcher and Judy continued their discussion, but with little energy and no resolution. The therapist had to remind Mr. Fletcher several times to restrain Irving from entering into the conversation, thus repeating his intervention on each occasion. Without Irving's participation, the conversation between the mother and Judy dribbled into awkward silence. The atmosphere in the room was stilted and strained. The father did as he was asked, but refused to register any enthusiasm for the task. Irving sulked, and the other children seemed bored, showing very clearly their intention to stay on the outside of the action. Near the end of the interview, the therapist summarized events, noting in particular how the family's flow and mood was radically altered when the father succeeded in stopping Irving from his "rescue operations." He assigned a modest task to the adults still living at home: the mother and Judy were to have three discussions about Judy's plans for next year. These were to be held in the evening. During this time, the father and Irving were to be in another room, watching TV or talking about nonessential topics. The whole family was asked to return for another interview.

Before the next interview occurred, Mrs. Fletcher called the therapist to say that Irving was worse than ever, that he had had several serious fights with Judy, a minor argument with Janice, and had stolen clothes from both of them. The therapist asked to speak to Mr. Fletcher, who confirmed what his wife had said. He also mentioned that he felt his wife was depressed, while he himself was very angry at Irving.

This clearly seemed a family in a crisis precipitated by the last interview and the homework task. The family's efforts now were to refocus on Irving, who was cooperating nicely through his misbehavior, and to return to the unhappy, but predictable balance that the family was in before entering treatment. The therapist insisted to Mr. Fletcher that the best course of action was to pursue the task they had agreed to, particularly that aspect requiring Irving to come to his father with his grievances about his sisters or his mother. The father was to assure Irving that he knew this would be difficult because he worried about his mother, lest she get "put out of a job." Furthermore, the therapist addressed the father's probable puzzlement and resistance to this notion by asking him to reassure his son (not himself) about it and to explain to Irving that "this may seem strange, but you worry too much about your mother. Leave that to me." The father agreed and actually seemed somewhat more accessible than before. He and the therapist chatted for a few minutes about other matters and agreed on the next appointment.

Crisis and Resistance

When the therapist foments a crisis in a family, creating a genuine turmoil by blocking the usual routes of behavioral exchange, there exists an opportunity for real change. A crisis atmosphere, however, can also engender great resistance to anything new happening. There is almost always a worsening of symptoms in the index patient; other members of the family begin to show signs of distress; and the structural innovation sought by the therapist seems a slender defense against the rising troubles of the family. No one is optimistic at these moments, and there is enormous pressure to return things to the status quo, especially through a renewed focus on the index patient. The family may directly indicate that the crisis behaviors are themselves an indication of how wrong the therapist has been and why the old routines were, after all, preferable to such widespread unhappiness. Previously, only one person was truly upset, but now the entire family is suffering, and so forth. It takes a confident therapist to ride this out; extra meetings may be required, as much to satisfy the therapist that life in the family is still manageable as to offer encouragement to the family. There are times when the pressure to change must be relieved, when the turmoil created by structural innovation goes beyond the opportunities of a normal family crisis and enters into a kind of runaway situation that benefits no one. Nevertheless, as with the results of any intervention, whether a task assignment during the interview or a major sequence interruption, the therapist must examine carefully the sources of the resistance before concluding that a temporary retreat is indicated.

At the next meeting, the Fletchers seemed dispirited and reluctant to join with the therapist in discussing all the unsettling events of the past week. All agreed that there had been more upsets than usual and that Mrs. Fletcher in particular had seemed depressed and listless. She had called her older daughters several times to complain about Irving and to express concerns about Judy's increasingly distant attitude. On one evening, Judy had not come home until well after midnight and the next day refused to say where she had been. When the therapist tried to activate his alliance with Mr. Fletcher, asking him to report on the tasks he was to oversee, Mr. Fletcher did so, but in a rather bland way. He had discussed with his wife her talks with Judy and found that nothing had changed there. He and Irving had, during the time of those talks, watched TV one night and talked briefly about sports another evening, but they forgot the assignment for the third evening. The therapist noted that they had succeeded in carrying out the spirit (the structure) of the task, even though the results (the content) had not seemed very positive. After this, he spent the remainder of the interview talking to the three oldest children, all of whom lived away from home. He chatted with them about apartments, rents, getting along with roommates, and about the emotional experience of the first few months away from home. When possible, he drew out features of their upbringing that were positive preparations for living on their own. All three showed real interest and energy in this discussion, in part because it was such a relief from the depression and demoralization of the group still living at home.

The shift to the older children had been intentional. It indicated that the crisis at home was real, but not of ominous proportions. Thus, there was freedom to turn the conversation to other matters, such as finding inexpensive apartments. The most notable features during this interview were (1) that much of the heat of Mrs. Fletcher's anger at Irving was gone, (2) that Irving did not respond to her nor get involved with Judy, and (3) that Mr. Fletcher seemed more concerned with his wife than had ever before been apparent.

Near the end of this interview, the therapist made three moves to continue the momentum for structural change. First, he explained to Judy and the mother that their initial conversations were a good step, but that Judy needed more information about living away from home. He asked Mrs. Fletcher's permission for Judy to spend one evening with Mary and one with Eileen to discuss their success in leaving home. She, of course, agreed to this, since her older daughters had already been publicly labeled as successful tributes to her parenting. Next, he warned Mr. Fletcher that his wife might seem more depressed in the next week, that she and Judy might have some flare-ups, and that he was to discuss these with her, but not to interfere beyond that. No comments at all were directed to Irving, and no one said anything about his behavior. Finally, an arrangement was made for the father to join the therapist in a school visit to hear first hand about Irving's difficulties at school. This extended the father's move into the parental subunit.

Working at the Interface

The word *interface* designates the temporal point and energetic force when information flows from one bounded system to another bounded system. It is the *interactional space* occupied by personal representatives of two different systems, each representative participating for the moment in the informational and purposive agendas of each system. The parent at a teacher–parent conference is operating at the interface between the family and the child's school. The parent represents both the values of the family and the parent's knowledge of the school system, balancing one against the other, sometimes in harmony, sometimes in conflict. The informational exchanges, verbal and nonverbal, betwen the parent and the teacher are described as interface behavior. When therapists choose those behaviors as a target for change, they may be described as "working at the interface." (See Fig. 8-1.)

We have in fact been speaking all along about interface work, since the very preference for structure rather than content compels us to examine the fate of systems in their surrounding contexts before knowing much about the specific psychological themes of the components of those systems. Our initial interests, for example, are in what actually happens when the children, one bounded system, transact business with the parents, a second bounded system. Actually, structural therapists always address behaviors at the interface between two systems. It is good diagnostic procedure to wonder at which subunit boundaries in interface with other subunit boundaries the family's troubles are located. Sometimes, the unit boundary where trouble occurs may be between the entire family unit and the surrounding neighborhood culture, as when a strongly ethnic family moves into an assimilated, nonethnic area, or when, as with the Fletchers, a working-class family finds housing in a predominantly upper-middle class, liberal neighborhood. Other times, the units involved are those within the larger family system. Locating the subunits involved and arranging to see the behavior that occurs at the interface between those units offers the therapist some notion of where change is needed.

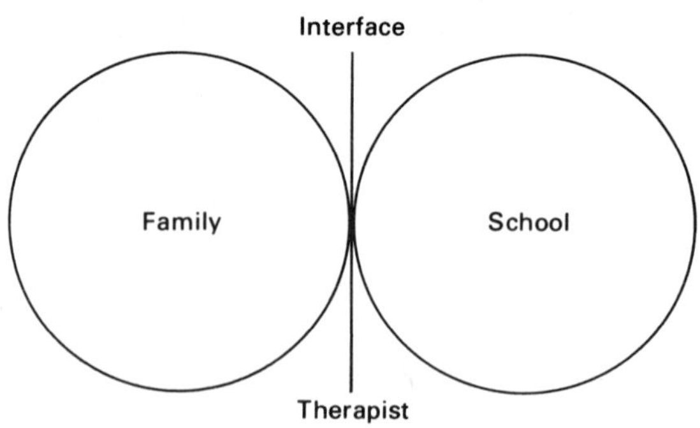

FIGURE 8-1. Diagram showing interface of adjacent systems.

The classic interfaces focused on are (1) between subunits within the family, (2) between family and school, (3) between family and courts, and (4) between the nuclear and extended family. Some structural work may consist of a good deal of attention to helping the different subsystems deal competently at the interface with other subsystems. This is often the case in helping poor, down-and-out families deal with the schools, courts, and housing agencies. Preparation for dealing at the interface between family and schools (or courts, etc.) may proceed through three phases:

1. *Rehearsal.* The therapist meets with key members of the family unit that will operate at the interface and offers help in how to deal effectively. Matters of group and individual communicational style may be addressed; some education in how the schools, courts, and other institutions actually operate may be necessary.
2. *Mediation.* Often the therapist will be present when the two units meet to transact business and will offer support, guidance, and therapeutic intervention on behalf of the client group that has been rehearsing. This is always the case when the units transacting business are within the family; it is generally the case when extrafamilial units are involved.
3. *Continuing contact.* Where there is some success and when behavior at the interface changes enough to allow both subunits to reach their goals and to deal cooperatively with each other, the therapist no longer need be present. Continuing contact between the units occurs without the therapist.

Throughout this effort, the therapist must not lose sight of the structural changes needed inside the family for it to recover from its current distress. For example, if one goal of therapy is to increase a peripheral father's involvement in the affairs of his children, and if this increased involvement is congruent with the family's values, then to have the mother deal competently at the interface between family and school is not helpful. The father needs to be rehearsed in coping with the school; his wife needs to be rehearsed in moving aside to allow him this new competency. Helping the family deal competently with the outside world requires that the therapist endorse and promote the family member whose participation in this role will also constitute some restructuring of the family itself.

During the third meeting with the Fletchers, certain changes were evident. Bob and Irving sat together, chatting about Bob's work. Mr. Fletcher sat between them and Janice, who was next to her mother. Mrs. Fletcher was flanked by Judy and her other two daughters. Irving began the meeting by reporting that there had been a big fight between his mother and Judy over her weekend plans and a date she had arranged. Two things were notable about this event: (1) Irving was now in the status of reporter rather than participant, and (2) he had actually stayed out of the fight at home. In fact, Irving's behavior had been quite good all week, a fact that was unnoticed until the therapist inquired. The greater concern was for the mother, who indeed seemed more distressed than when treatment began, and for Judy, who was becoming more defiant in her plans to leave home. Mr. Fletcher had not really spoken to his wife about her distress (as requested by the therapist), although it was quite evident to him. The older sisters reported pleasant meetings with Judy, but otherwise declined to participate in the interview. Bob was silent as usual, though clearly in greater contact with Irving than were other family members. The focus of distress seemed to be Mrs. Fletcher and, in an indirect way, her husband, who was unable to respond to her. At this point, the therapist suggested he see only the parents for several sessions, not because of their marital issues (which had never been part of the initial contract), but because they were both weary and a little dispirited over the many problems in the family. The therapist emphasized his view that in fact many things were getting under control. He added, however, that the prospect of Judy's leaving seemed to change things for Mrs. Fletcher, and this was a concern for the grownups—not the children, especially not Irving—to address. They agreed to a "couples only" visit for the next week.

Stage 4: Shifting to the Parents Alone

A good deal of family therapy seems to evolve itself rather quickly into marital therapy. There are good reasons for this, and one must be impressed by the ample evidence that reveals that many psychological forces are present when parents involve their children as expressions of their difficulties with each other. Broadly viewed, the child either becomes, as Minuchin (1974) has called it, a kind of "conflict avoidance circuit," which allows the parents to continue their marriage in good-natured, but deceptive harmony, united in their anger and dismay at their rotten child; or the child is involved in a deadly cross-generational alliance with one parent against the other. Neither place is good for a child, and a therapist naturally wishes to get the child out of there as soon as possible (or to detriangulate the child, as the jargon goes). This view of the psychology of childhood disorders continues to be transactional, though it implicitly relies on rather traditional notions of displacement and projective identification. Procedures for change can stay in the realm of structural therapy regardless of these underlying psychological presumptions. Given this perspective, it is not surprising that so many family therapists move quickly to the marital subsystem as the focus of change.

This shift merits some cautionary remarks. First, therapists should not make this shift too soon by calling on the husband and wife to settle their differences before they have had a chance to improve their parenting behaviors. Parents seldom respond to an invitation for family therapy except as worried parents; they do not ask for marital counseling and would find comments on their marriage to be gratuitous and even impolite. Whether or not they know about the issues in their marriage is beside the point: they may know and *not* wish to address them directly. This avoidance, in fact, can be of tremendous advantage to the therapist who recognizes that in a land of isomorphic transformations, the structures of parenting may be read as metaphors for the structures of marriage. If the therapist is content to help them improve and alter their cooperation as parents, certain issues of the marriage are inevitably addressed. For this reason, it may be more useful to continue family meetings that involve the children and that offer the grownups a chance to practice new parenting skills than to plunge the parents into the anxiety of their marital problems.

Second, shifting focus to the couple should not be viewed as the final stage of treatment. As in work with any other subsystem, the therapist keeps in mind the larger family goals of change and how the renovated parental unit can fit back into those goals. Seeing the couple is not something to do in anticipation of never seeing the children again. Whatever does or does not change in their marital roles, the spouses must ultimately also continue their daily contact with their children. In this way, the spouses are simply another subunit in the family and must be responsive to the larger design for family functioning that has evolved.

Third, work with the spouses, even when it is specifically about their marriage, can be successful for the larger family, though no change may occur between the husband and wife. That is, since a major impetus behind this shift is to help free the children from entanglements between their parents, a therapist can educate the parents to behave in new ways while assuring them that they need not alter the interpersonal distance in their marriage. Often parents will arrive at just such a position on their own, despite the therapist's efforts to improve their marriage. Parents, in short, can be helped to find new and better ways of dealing with their children while simply finding new strategies to continue their marital struggles. If they must triangulate in a third entity to pursue their fights, then it is better for that entity to be a job, a pet, or an in-law than one of their children.

Finally, these cautionary remarks are not meant to discourage the prospect of straightforward marital therapy. Many couples who as concerned parents enter therapy often ask of their own accord for help with marital issues. In those instances, the therapist proceeds according to whatever brand of marital work he or she prefers; there is nothing technically new that structural family therapy has to offer about couples counseling. Structural therapy only helps therapists know why at this juncture in altering the system they would be well advised to see the couple and how to fit the couple holon back into the larger systems picture.

Actually, Mr. and Mrs. Fletcher missed the next appointment, an event suggesting the extent of their ambivalence about appearing together. It was also characteristic of this therapist that he failed to prepare the family adequately for another staging intervention; as a result, subsequent appointments were often missed. At any rate, he phoned the next day and learned that each parent independently had forgotten the appointment until that evening. He set another time and advised that they help Judy keep her appointments with the older sisters and that Irving continue to register his family complaints only with his father.

The next week, during the first interview with the couple, the therapist learned of a long and difficult marital history that centered around two major complaints. The wife complained of her husband's periodic trouble with drinking, though it had never threatened his rather successful work life; she also accused him of "improper" behavior toward the older daughters, especially when they were younger. The sexual implication was clear. He furiously denied this, and she did not press the issue, saying only that she suspected it. Her attitude toward him and whatever real transgressions he may have made helped explain the current aloofness of his daughters toward him.

On his part, he complained about his wife's remoteness from him, especially her overinvolvement with her own mother, whom she spoke to nearly every day. Until now, the full extent of Mrs. Fletcher's tie to her mother was not clear; now she discussed her deep devotion to her mother, noting that her father died early in her life and that she was raised by her mother and her sister, and her growing depression as her mother became elderly and infirm. Her mother had declined a good deal in just the last two years, after Mary and Eileen had left home. Now it seemed clear why the mother was so sensitive to Judy's leaving home—it coincided with the anticipated loss of her own mother. With no female buffer, Mrs. Fletcher would be left with only her husband and Janice, assuming Irving also left in a few years.

There was another side to all this. They had loved each other, married, and raised a family that was unremarkable and reasonably well until the recent events that brought them to treatment. They had been married for many years and looked forward to some pleasures of no longer raising so many children. It clearly was a mixed case: they had their complaints about each other, but they also showed little motivation for a radical alteration in their relationship. In addition, each had individual issues of long-standing that had not been solved in the marriage; actually, they had found spouses and developed a pattern that conformed to their individual neuroses. The wife, unfamiliar with men, found a husband who was often distant, drinking, and very caught up in his work, and who, for the most part, did not intrude into her alliances with the daughters. The exceptions were those times when, under the influence of alcohol, he angered his wife by becoming overinvolved with his daughters. As for Mr. Fletcher, a man not given to much emotional expression and often unsure of how to be inside the family (his greater competence being in the world), it was quite to his advantage to have a wife who took over and left him in a peripheral position. How should a therapist, interested in family change, regard these individual problems?

Individual Issues and Family Structure

There are always psychological factors that precede and supercede the development of a new nuclear family life. This is obviously the case with the partners who start the family. It is less apparent with the children who arrive, though each new member has tempermental and energetic features not only undetermined by family forces, but also very little modified over time. Mrs. Fletcher, for example, has apparently always retained special sensitivities about being more safe with women than with men, yet she helped create a family and, over the years did a reasonable job of allowing the children to grow up without devastating enmeshments in her neurotic concerns. Even Irving was not terribly handicapped and, moreover, his difficulties had as much to do with a rather distant father as with his mother. Mrs. Fletcher's incipient depression will remain as a constant feature, as will Irving's possibly intractable learning problems.

Whether the entire family could be mobilized to help either person or whether it should even be involved are probably questions for endless debate. Family structures can evolve just so far and only at a rate commensurate with maintaining the system in a healthy balance between growth and stasis and between the promotion of individual diversity and collective unity. Undoubtedly, some individual problems can improve within the regulatory settings of the family system. Others will require solution by referral to other settings, such as individual psychotherapy, where the system limits are different and where the settings for growth and change are at a rate and level permitting the kind of development that may be impossible to achieve working only within the family. Family structure, and the therapy of family structure, is a powerful setting within which considerable individual change occurs; it is also a setting whose *immediate* possibilities are rather quickly exhausted. At that point, the system will probably continue at a new level until events—either those of the natural life cycle or those from the surrounding culture, which are unexpected—

precipitate another evolutionary move. When individual issues cannot find resolution within the temporal and energetic settings of the family system, involvement in other therapies seems helpful.

The Fletchers met several times just as a couple. During these times, they discussed some serious differences about their children. Although, for example, Irving continued to keep a new, low profile with his sister and mother, Mrs. Fletcher continued to describe him as a potential source of trouble, a person who, like her husband, *might* get out of control even though currently well behaved. This, and other equations of her husband and son, were pointed out to her. She was encouraged to drop Irving from the battle, but not necessarily to change her convictions about her husband. Naturally, as her husband became more involved with Irving, taking his side at times, Mrs. Fletcher found it difficult to make this separation. What turned the tide for her was the therapist's persistent focus on getting Mr. Fletcher to take a sympathetic stance toward his wife's feelings of impending loss of her mother and, shortly, of Judy. Here, the therapist frankly banked on his alliance with Mr. Fletcher, since Mrs. Fletcher did not initially reinforce his efforts. While struggles over how to respond to the children at home continued, the parents were also reminded to carry on with the new regimes of letting Judy spend more time with her older sisters, set her own curfews, and date more. Mrs. Fletcher also agreed that her husband could continue to be the person to whom Irving went with both his school and home complaints. The single concrete task assigned to the couple was this: whenever Mrs. Fletcher became upset with Judy or worried about her mother, she was to mention this to her husband, who would listen sympathetically, but *not* question her about her concerns or in any way require that she have any additional contact with him. This task gave them some link and deflected the tendency to be overinvolved with the children. It also communicated respect for Mrs. Fletcher's anxiety about her husband and his preference for emotional quiet. With these few accomplishments well in hand, the therapist suggested they adjourn the meetings for a month to see how well the family would do entirely on its own.

The Last Stage: The Parents and Children Living at Home

During the recess, Mr. Fletcher had called the therapist several times to report on the family. Since there were no pressing issues, they held off meeting for another month. At this final meeting, the therapist asked for only those family members who were actually living at home—the parents and the three children. By this time, there seemed no clear reason for the family to continue therapy, since the original complaints about Irving had either subsided or were being handled. His difficulties at home had virtually stopped, and he no longer seemed bad or peculiar; however, his school difficulties had not improved, except in one respect. His clashes with his male teachers had definitely stopped, although they were replaced by some difficulty with his peers, who still viewed him as somewhat immature and hence available for teasing. His academic problems persisted, and by now, he had accumulated a poor school record for six years. His learning problems were substantial, and his father had scheduled another meeting between himself, the teacher, and Irving. He and Irving were tentatively determined to help him finish high school and then enlist in the Army, as his brother had done. The plans were optimistic, but Irving's prospects seemed limited. On the other hand, he was clearly happy about his improved position at home. He enjoyed greater contact with his father and a vastly improved relationship with his sister, whose early exit from the home he supported. Mrs. Fletcher and Judy still had some tough moments together, but with Irving out of the immediate conflict, their differences did not get sealed over, and they were feeling able to deal with them. Judy spent more time with her older sisters and had enrolled in a secretarial training school for the next school term. The parents, who met with the therapist alone for a short while, seemed clear about what the children were doing and in general agreement about parenting. They did not report any greater contact with each other, except occasional conversations about Mrs. Fletcher's concern over her mother, who was undergoing another serious illness. They also shared with the therapist some worries about Janice, who seemed more out of hand since things had been settled with the older children. The therapist agreed with their assessment that Janice had always had to take a back seat because she was so much younger and so good; now they assumed Janice felt it was her turn to be listened to, and the parents thought that was right. Clearly, they could continue the union as cooperative parents around Janice. Equally clear was the opportunity for Janice now to become overinvolved with her mother, a danger the therapist spelled out for them. How the spouses would finally deal with each other once all the children had left home was anyone's guess. They would probably do no worse than most.

The family had been seen for a total of 17 times (including the school visit) over a period of six months.

Part III

LOOKING AT STRUCTURE

Chapter 9

The Structural Advantage

The Fletcher family fared well enough to be considered a successful treatment endeavor, and at this point, the beginning family therapist may now have some clear ideas as to how that happened. With equal measures of effort and good fortune, the beginning therapist will have begun to acquire some mastery of the fundamental tenants of systems theory and of structural therapy. But there naturally remain unanswered questions about structural family therapy. What are its best uses? What are its limits? Why is it so hard to learn the language of systems? What is the relationship of structural family therapy to other theories of therapy?

These are the concluding concerns of this book and the focus of this last chapter. Throughout this final discussion, one may recognize that there are domains of phenomena not even addressed, or poorly addressed, by systems theory and structural therapy; this makes comparison to other theories of change both easier and more difficult. It is easier, because certain traditional psychological constructs, such as "motivation," are simply not of central concern to systems theory; therefore, no comparison can meaningfully be made to, say, psychoanalysis, which directs a good deal of attention to issues of motivation. But the task of comparison to other theories is also rendered more difficult when parallel comparisons are not possible and when the competing theories of change do not even consider the same data, which would then be differently interpreted according to one's theoretical perspective. In these instances, we can simply note whatever beginning efforts are being made to achieve some similarity of experiential focus, as, for example, in the recent efforts of systems theorists to direct more attention to the phenomonology of individual experience. To begin discussion of these several questions, one may broadly divide the topics into those most associated with (1) theories of behavior and then with (2) issues of actual clinical practice.

THE STRUCTURAL APPROACH AND THEORIES OF BEHAVIOR

The domains of experience best addressed by structural family therapy are those given prominence by a general systems theory of behavior. We will review that theory briefly and in such a way that one gains a synopsis of the central topics covered in all the preceding chapters. These topics are the areas of concern included within the structural approach. But some items of experience will seem omitted or only faintly recognized by the systems paradigm, though, by contrast, these same items are the core concerns of other theories of change. These contrasts will be examined when the more psychodynamic theories of family process are discussed and when we review recent efforts to expand the domains of data included within a general systems view of human activity.

Fundamentals of Systems Theory and Structural Therapy

One might arrive at some structural techniques without a notion of systems, but the general systems paradigm is what gives theoretical coherence to structural family therapy. This systems paradigm is a biological and cybernetic model that describes the interrelated evolution of parts into an increasingly complex, adaptive whole. The whole, when it is a living system, modifies its adaptive exchanges with the environment through a series of mutually causal feedback loops. The circularity inherent in feedback loops creates a model of conditions for life and for change that goes beyond traditional, linear notions of cause and effect. Because the living system, from biological cell to social group, is subdivided into interrelated parts, the resulting totality constitutes an environmental context, or surrounding, for a particular part. This depiction permits a new conception of psychological metaphors—such as "self" and "mind." It suggests that these metaphorical "parts" be viewed as interactive phenomena, not as "things" historically hatched within an impervious individual body. A theory of development of self-in-context suggests a therapy that modifies the context-around-self. Indeed, one fundamental premise of structural family therapy lies in the belief that if one modifies the interactional context, changes in individual behavior will follow.

From the systems paradigm and from this basic premise about change—that alterations in context create change in the parts—Minuchin and his colleagues developed their views of normal and pathological family development. From this developmental perspective, the family, in accordance with the rules for living systems, must consist of some subsystems, each one with definite boundary properties. In living systems, there must also be hierarchical arrangements among the parts and the subsystems. There is also the formation of alliances and coalitions among the parts, sometimes within a subsystem and sometimes across subsystem boundaries. Normal families show a capacity to rotate these alliances and coalitions so that no one family member is pinned forever in one grouping; yet the family also provides for the stable, relatively enduring "boundedness" of some of its subsystems, such as the marital unit. This alternation of flexibility with stability and of the opportunity for novelty with the assurance of some constancy characterizes the adaptive living system. Nonadaptive or pathological systems show many of the opposite traits. They are rigid in their coalitions and alliances, regardless of the content issue. Boundaries between subsystems are either too open or too closed. Hierarchies are inverted. People are forced into triangular arrangements, and the larger environmental context has a diminishingly corrective effect on family behavior.

Structural family therapy as a theory attends to these fundamental facets of the living system—boundaries, hierarchies, information exchanges with the outside world, and so on. The therapist actually directs attention to these phenomena in clinical cases. Therapy proceeds as a series of intervention strategies consistent with the underlying theory. The first of these strategies appears as the therapist joins the family and begins to make a structural diagnosis. Structural family therapy emphasizes the act of joining as an act of diagnosis. Moving into the life of a family is an active event and has the status of an intervention. How the family responds to this intrusion reveals the outlines of its patterned functioning. These outlines point the way to the substantive structural arrangements most characteristic of the family at this point in time. Joining activity may occur from a relatively disengaged position, as when the therapist directs the family in some enactment of its core problems. From this position, the therapist makes observations of how the family behaves once it is in motion. Or the therapist may join from more of an inside position, accommodating to the apparent structural preferences of the family, showing sympathy and understanding, and refraining from direct challenges. In this position, the therapist learns what it feels like to be converted to the family's way and picks up the tempo and mood of family life while retaining the ability to observe as well as to feel. Throughout the initial diagnostic phase and treatment itself, there is always a clear appreciation that the therapist's presence, style, and direction constitute forces that may change the family structure.

Through the experience of joining and the gathering of impressions about family life, the therapist arrives at a structural diagnosis. This diagnosis is a series of propositions in words and diagrams about (1) the alliances and coalitions within the family; (2) the boundary properties of the total family unit and its subsystems; (3) the hierarchical distribution of executive power; and (4) the key interactional sequences that are the operational source of these abstracted structures and that give experiential meaning to them. Above all, the structural diagnosis is an hypothesis about the systemic interaction between the total family context and the symptomatic behaviors of individual members. To make a structural diagnostic statement is to say something about the way people are positioned for contact with each other and with other subsystems. This diagnosis does not prevent the therapist from making corollary assumptions about events hard to observe or verify, such as the inner feelings and wishes of individual family members, but it does make those assumptions peripheral in drawing up plans about what to do. Structural therapists argue that matters of internal motivation and emotional readiness for a new type of relational contact may eventually move to the forefront, but not until there have been successful alterations of the structural positions of each family member.

Data for a structural diagnosis come primarily from observations of family behavior during the interview. Quite secondarily, data come from a family's report of behavior and from a family's history. Within the interview, the therapist makes use of spontaneous behaviors, directed enactments among family members, and the consequences of rearranging the total context, as in meetings with smaller subsystems of the family. On the basis of such data, a diagnostic hypothesis is made, and tentative plans for treatment are formed.

In order to test a structural hypothesis, the therapist needs to involve the family in a shared view of the problem. A family usually enters treatment with a rather linear notion of the trouble—namely, that one person, the symptom bearer, is controlling the entire family. Minuchin has been emphatic about the need to challenge this assumption and to help the family arrive at a redefinition of the presenting problem. This redefinition helps the family shift to the idea that the family group sustains the troubled individual. The redefinition needs to be plausible and not blaming; otherwise, the family will not return. A redefinition of the presenting symptom is only a restatement of the problem in terms of those recurrent family transactions that make possible the continuation of the symptomatic behavior. It is not a dismissal of the symptom, but a reframing of its meaning for the total system. Properly done, a redefinition is, in actuality, a restructuring intervention into the family's prevailing life patterns. A good redefinition implicitly carries with it the other essential features of beginning treatment: a statement about who in the family would be most important in reaching that goal (not necessarily the entire family) and an outline of the stages in which treatment will proceed. When these matters are clearly developed, treatment is already well underway.

The theoretical plan for structural change and treatment involves the notion of induced crisis or systems instability as a step in systems transformation. The classic interventions associated with structural family therapy are designed both to induce crisis and to support the durability of new structures. Intervention strategies all emerge from one perspective: initial attention to structure, not to psychological content. The strategies most associated with the structural approach are the following: (1) the staging of symptom-oriented interventions in the overall flow of the treatment plan; (2) the interruption of dysfunctional alliances and coalitions; (3) the correction of hierarchical problems; (4) the observation and alteration of critical, pathologic behavioral sequences that maintain a stagnant homeostasis; (5) the assignment of tasks, both within the interview and at home; and (6) the offering of descriptions of the family's behavioral process. As the family changes, these interventions lose the form of identifiable contributions from the therapist and instead become an indistinguishable part of the family's usual way of living.

In summary, the systems paradigm and the structural therapy derived from it emphasize the transcendence of the whole over its parts; yet, through the principle of circular causality, that whole remains also defined by the activity of these parts. The paradigm encourages attention to observable behaviors that occur in the here and now, and in this regard, it is ahistorical theory. Therapeutic endeavors are initially, and even predominately, addressed to the behavioral exchanges at the boundaries of interfacing units rather than to suppositions about events going on inside a single unit, such as an individual family member. Restructuring both the myths and the phenomena of everyday life is the primary goal of therapy, and it is the job of the therapist to create opportunities for such changes to occur.

Throughout its relatively short life as an influential theory of behavior and change, general systems theory has always been compared to psychodynamic theories of individual behavior and to psychoanalytic theory in particular. Why there are such persistent comparisons, and such persistent efforts to integrate the two different paradigms, are questions to be addressed. But first, a brief outline of the psychoanalytic paradigm needs to be drawn, so that one might sense at least the shadow of the theory that has so dominated psychological thinking for over a half-century.

Fundamentals of Psychoanalytic Theory and Therapy

Until about 1950, the evolution of personality and the regulatory principles governing human activity were largely drawn from the paradigm of psychoanalytic psychology. The specific propositions of this model were diverse, complicated, and substantiated primarily by clinical anecdote. It was preeminently a model of individual development and behavior, a model in which past and present exchanges with real people were studied through the verbal reports, given retrospectively, about the internal images of those actual behaviors. In this way, a person's internal life became the proper unit for both scientific inquiry and clinical intervention. Here lay what Rabkin (1970) called the "inner space imponderables," those affects, memories, and fleeting thoughts that cannot be seen directly, but are pondered only through the reports of the person who contains them. Indeed, much of the language of this paradigm suggested a "container-ingredient" theory of human experience: the skin-encased "self" is the container for an infinitude of ingredients—anger, lust, anxiety, warring dreams, and peaceful hopes.

Naturally, such ingredients must be organized if mental entropy was not to prevail. The psychoanalytic model provided organizing rules through postulation of overriding mental structures, such as ego, superego, and id, and the presence of dynamic, propelling "forces," such as the unconscious and the conscious mind, terms that designate both a kind of "place" and a process.

As Roy Schafer pointed out (1978), however, such organizational apparatus needed to be driven if the human machine was to do more than lie about, lost in an orderly lassitude of internal images; hence, the importance of libido, a biologically rooted energetic force, frequently sexualized (though as frequently not), that could propel the individual through life. Psychological motives and urges were given the status of propulsive entities that brought about actual behaviors; for example, a *person* did not behave conflictually, but the person's *mental processes* did. The imagery and metaphor of a machine was unavoidably evoked by these propositions, a ". . . machine that will not work in the absence of properly applied propulsive forces . . . [found] in the biological process of the organism" (Schafer, 1978, p.195).

Other defining features of this paradigm then became necessary. If there are structures that organize these interior processes and propulsive energies, which are themselves regulated by routine assignment and reassignment to various psychic areas of the larger psychological territory, then there must be some hierarchical principals governing the development of these regulatory processes. Notions of developmental time now appeared, suggesting that indeed the psychological birth of the human being was an unfolding process, with some psychic agencies appearing before others. This process, in turn, introduced the metaphor of "depth," which suggested that what was developed earlier in life was also "deeper"—that is, less accessible through intentional recall and, perhaps for this reason, awarded greater aesthetic and psychological significance than those psychic events and developmental structures that emerged later in life. The metaphor of depth perpetuated a mechanistic notion of man, as though there existed a vertical dimension of psychic layers, a kind of interior village that required a psychological archeology in order for the total history of the person to be reconstructed.

Finally, intimately bound to the notions of development, hierarchy, depth, and vertical layering, the psychoanalytic model, unlike the systems model, was persistently historical in its temporal orientation. In part because of this and in part because of the mechanistic principles that characterize the basic suppositions, psychoanalysis was firmly bound by a linear notion of cause and effect. What comes first greatly determines what comes later; what was done can seldom be undone, at least with regard to the general patternings of behavior known as character. This is in marked contrast to the premise of circular causality in the systems model.

In spite of this emphasis on a person as propelled by a biologically based energy, psychoanalysis did not presuppose an environmental vacuum. Although beginning with the internal life of the individual, the model included much about the interpersonal context surrounding the person. This information, however, was gathered in a manner consistent with the paradigm's major premises—specifically, that the outer world was best known through one's inner account of it, that account being retrievable and reported primarily through verbal recall. This, again, contrasts with the preference of the systems theorist for *observed behavior* rather than reports about behavior. It was one of the ironies of psychoanalysis that it consistently drew attention to the vital importance of the individual's membership in groups (family, clan, tribe, and larger cultural setting), yet was equally consistent in understanding such membership only as filtered through the focal vision of a single protagonist, the analysand who, through introspection, told about the workings of culture on an individual mind. It was left to others—such as anthropologists, and later, systems therapists—to observe the daily routines and random behavioral exchanges that made up the individual's behavior in culture groups.

Summing the Comparisons

On the level that most clinicians use theory, there are obvious differences between the systems and the psychodynamic paradigm; whether or not, at some greater level of abstraction, these differences are reconcilable remains to be demonstrated, an achievement not yet convincingly made. Certainly in the realm of daily clinical effort, the differences are clear: there are contrasting models of causality, dramatically different data bases, striking contrasts in techniques for joining (the analyst is neutral; the structural therapist is leading), considerable variation in the locus of a therapeutic intervention (inside the individual versus inside the interpersonal context), and evident differences in the use of historical versus present time. Given such lack of fit, why indeed does one bother trying to force the paradigms to fit together in some way, perhaps in a continuing search for some unified theory of behavior? Why not settle for multiple versions of experiential reality and accept that sometimes the psychodynamic paradigm seems best suited to guide one's therapeutic efforts and, other times, the systems paradigm is a superior guide? Why, in short, distract oneself from the potentials of a systems-structural viewpoint through interruptive cross reference to the psychodynamic perspective? There are at least two obvious reasons. The first concerns an apparently natural reluctance on one's part to make the leap to a systems model, and the second reason is created by difficulties within structural theory itself.

A CHANGE OF MIND

The perception of superordinate structures may be possible, but where, the beginning therapist wonders, is room for the life of the inner person? Indeed, for all the obvious clinical power of structural family therapy concepts and for all the allure of systems theory, there remains for most therapists great difficulty in mastering this newer paradigm of behavior. A good deal of that difficulty is actually the reluctance to change one's mind about what is *really* important in daily experience. Family systems therapy in general has found it difficult to change the minds of therapists who are surrounded by the constraints of individual psychology. Structural family therapy is no exception, despite the obvious intentions of Minuchin to award some centrality to individual experience. Intentions aside, any teacher of the structural approach will admit that it is the rare student who very easily learns to "see" systems. On the contrary, beginning family therapists find it difficult to change their minds about what is important in behavior, at least if such a change minimizes individual life events.

Resistance to the systems paradigm is not only a fault of how that paradigm has been promoted by its advocates, but is powerfully rooted in the phenomenal reality of every human being. This resistance to a change-of-mind lies in one's experience of oneself as a bounded, individual entity, a kind of skin-encased unit that encloses a continually active mass of sensations, pulsations, associations, fantasies, images, dreams, and thoughts. It is difficult to require, as apparently systems theory might require, that one minimize this daily stream of intensely personal events simply because a newer theory has not yet made good use of them. If anything, such a requirement seems a reflection of the poor quality of the theory, certainly not of the thinness of one's private life. One seldom, if ever, experiences oneself as primarily moved through life by the intersecting vectors of systemic field forces. On the other hand, one is quite ready to claim that last night's dream, this morning's waking fantasy, and one's current thoughts are indeed the very stuff of life. These emotional, cognitive, and imagistic events are all internal, at least in one's *experience* of them. From this perspective, it often appears to new therapists that a systems theory asks them to view as nonessential the very experiences that seem so intensely and quintessentially human, experiences whose phenomenal reality is inescapable and whose presence makes one unique among animals. To exchange the phenomenal richness of inner life for the abstractions of systems theory seems a poor trade.

Moreover, while people are reluctant to locate the source of interpersonal difficulties as within themselves, they are even more reluctant to give up a primary focus on one's interior drama in exchange for the invisible forces of cultural context. Thus, the psychoanalytic model offered the best way of conceptualizing what makes up our consciousness of self. If not always convincing and if even occasionally shocking in some of its propositions about humankind, the model's labyrinthine complexity certainly matched that of our personal introspections. There was something grand and restorative in contemplating the awesome magnificence of the psychic machinery that psychoanalysis placed inside human beings. In contrast to the mechanistic theories of American behaviorism, the psychoanalytic paradigm often made intuitive sense; it gave order to the stream of mental life we all experienced, and it promised the correlation of psychological life with the discoveries of biology and physics—sciences the exactness of which had long been the envy of students of human behavior. And with regard to change, one would continue to be propelled by private inner forces, but with these more thoroughly understood and made explicit, then surely one's life in public contexts would improve.

PRIVATE SELVES, PUBLIC STRUCTURES

One's natural reluctance to switch from self to system is made even greater by an historical error within the teaching of structural family therapy. The error was a readiness to dismiss the internal life of individuals as too associated with the older, psychodynamic paradigm and therefore antithetical to the data requirements of general systems theory. It is important to understand that systems theory does not itself require the exclusion of the data of individual, interior experience; however, the early didactic emphasis in structural family therapy implicitly forbade making good use of such data. In a sense, structural family therapy has failed to be a fully cybernetic theory of human behavior because of its reluctance to include fully the phenomenology of individual experience in the behavioral loops comprising a family's experiential context. This failure would seem to be rectified by the work of Minuchin and Fishman (1981). They made complete statements about the importance of the individual in family process, gave individuals the same theoretical status as other subunits of a family, and discussed, however briefly, the development of "mind" and "self" as systems phenomena. (See below for a fuller discussion of this effort.) Clearly, their intention was to include the individual, but in actuality, it was too simple. Naturally, in theory, individuals must be included as part of the system. While the system may be a superordinate organization, it nonetheless is composed of "some things," and those things are, in part, individual human beings. So naturally, the theory of family systems must include human beings. Hardly startling, it is a step. There the process generally stops. In actual practice and in most of the writing on structural family therapy, there is, in fact, little attention paid to *how* precisely the alterations of individual, internal states then reverberate back through the system. Thus, the consistent and careful attention to changing family structure (and hence, presumably, the inner life of the individual family members) is not complemented by attention to techniques for affecting the interior life of individuals. The short-sighted systems theorist seems content to show the effects of context on character, but is quite unwilling to complete the circle, as logically required by an organismic paradigm, and to show how changed individuals now affect, in turn, the context in which they live. To show the individual either as "effect" or "cause" would require gathering information about interior life, a task difficult to imagine without falling back into the traditional tactics of linear, psychoanalytic psychology. Hence, the circle is never completed, and the structural therapist is forced to settle for a linear two-step instead of the complete dance.

SOME SOLUTIONS

Solutions, some less successful than others, have appeared. Among psychoanalytic family theorists, many have simply preempted systems theory and family process studies by noting, in naive ways, that Freud anticipated most of what family theory is all about; for example, Freud often spoke of family forces and clearly recognized their centrality in character formation (Sanders, 1979). Such efforts at an integration of the two paradigms demonstrated a misunderstanding of both the premises and the opportunities of systems theory. Other theorists have postulated some internal dynamic that serves as a kind of "missing link" between the individual and the interpersonal system. For example, Kantor (1980) has spoken of a "critical identity image" as linking the interior self with the interpersonal system. Slipp (1980) gave similar status to his notion of "symbiotic survival pattern." These links seem burdened with all the antiquated theories of energy and metaphysics characteristic of psychoanalysis in its earlier phases. Although such approaches have given credibility to transactional systems, they have confused what works clinically with a meaningful description of individuals, which is also theoretically congruent with the data requirements of systems theory.

A more substantial effort to account for private lives within public systems has been made by the proponents of traditional psychodynamic family therapy. Theorists like Bowen (1978), Nagy (1973), and Framo (1970) have consistently spoken of systems principles while providing a glue between the parts that has been mostly made up of psychoanalytic constructs. Thus, while their integrative effort was sophisticated, there remain important differences between them and the interpretation of systems theory represented by structural therapists. The latter continue to emphasize process, ecology, and the contemporaneous behavioral transactions that maintain symptoms. The psychodynamic family therapists often give their most careful attention to matters of psychological content, to the genesis of symptoms, to reports of historical antecedents of symptomatic behavior, and then to the removal of these problems through interpretation of the often unconscious forces they believe are reflected in the symptoms. Their approaches give considerable weight to the phenomena of individual experience, but as with other such solutions, they falter in the conceptualization of these experiences in ways that are compatible with general systems theory.

Minuchin was well aware of this problem and has given it increased attention. His "solution" deserves careful review since it represents the most recent attempt by structuralists to conceptualize individual experience in a way that is consistent with the premises of systems theory. He and Fishman, in their 1981 work, have shown a consistent regard for the view that a person can be both a whole and a part of some larger system, but that the experience of oneself as a separate whole is still unalterably linked with the forces of mutuality and reciprocity between a part and its context. According to them, "Inner self is entwined inextricably with social context: they form a single unit. To separate one from the other is . . . to stop the music in order to hear it more clearly. It disappears!" (p.12). They have objected to any epistemology that suggests a dichotomy between the individual as a self-contained whole and the self as part of a larger context. For Minuchin and Fishman, the "self" is only a "self-in-context," and any experience of separateness from context is an illusion created by selective focus. Psychoanalysis, they have argued, has created just such an illusion, that of an internalized context where the drama of daily life is a dance among introjects of past relationships. An interpersonal, or systems approach, on the contrary, keeps the organizing context outside; this circumscribes one's individual freedom without challenging one's individuality. It is clearly the work of a systems-oriented family therapy to expand one's personal notion of self to include the reality of complementary relations with other members of the family. Instead of an "I" view of the world, each person learns to observe the other person as a context for the self. From this perspective, the therapist says, "Help the other person change, which will change yourself as you relate to him and will change both of you within the holon" (Minuchin & Fishman, 1981, p.197).

The critical link between individual and system is to imagine an endless, circular process in which selected aspects of the individual self are called into play and reinforced; in this strengthened state, they then serve to call forth reciprocal attributes in another member of the family group. According to Minuchin and Fishman:

> Specific transactions with other people elicit and reinforce those aspects of the individual's personality that are appropriate to the context. The individual, in turn, affects the other people who interact with her in certain ways because her responses have elicited and reinforced their responses. There is a circular, continuous process of mutual affecting and reinforcing, which tends to maintain a fixed pattern. At the same time, both individual and context have the capacity for flexibility and change (p.14).

These theoretical efforts to explain individual variance while remaining loyal to a systems paradigm seems promising. Furthermore, Minuchin and Fishman have derived some concrete clinical moves from this viewpoint.

For example, they may frame one person's behavior in terms of an interaction rather than as an attribute of the self. In response to a husband who says, "I feel bored," they might ask: "What does your wife do to bore you?" The emphasis is shifted from an internal "I" to a transactional "we." In the end, it is a matter of focus and perspective. There are many feelings and thoughts that can be reframed in a transactional way and just as many that elude such redefinition. Structural family therapy chooses to focus on what can be reframed and to leave alone those internal events whose mystery must be explored through different methods.

Whether or not the efforts of Minuchin and Fishman to create a plausible link between individual and system will be honored remains to be seen. But unlike other integrative efforts, their explanatory concepts were consistent with the basic premises of systems theory. One is not required to mix models or to preempt the systems viewpoint by locating its analogy in some early writings of Freud. How to make sense of our interior life will no doubt continue to occupy both practitioners and researchers of family systems theory. So much of our interior experience is rich and laden with layers of meaning that a simple recasting of this material into the language of interpersonal context seems only partially satisfactory. Yet the effort of Minuchin and Fishman was clearly in the right direction and might prove easier to use if one took seriously that all such therapeutic reframing is, among other things, a matter of language use. Linguistic communications can be essential data in a general systems theory of behavior.

If one attends to language, then general systems theory has itself provided one way to observe the integration of individual experience with family process. That is, all living systems need constantly to transmit information across subunit boundaries in order to regulate the alternating processes of growth and stability, of diversity and unity. This transmission process is a communication about the relationship of one living system to another, whether that system is an individual or a subunit of individuals. This communication process can be observed through the study of spoken language and additional nonverbal signals. Language is an experience and a form of data completely congruent with a general systems model of behavior, in part because it is utterly contemporaneous, occurring always in the here and now. These language activities are not simply a medium, an ether through which are transmitted the colorful contents of our inner life. They are not a cloak around the body of inner experiences. Language activities are the primary interpersonal event; in a sense, they create the public event and, in so doing, create the relationship of the speaker to the listener. It is this linguistic reality, this arranging and regulating of relationships among family members, that constitutes the data one can observe from a systems perspective.

An emphasis on interpersonal reality as a linguistic phenomena is consistent with the view held by Minuchin and Fishman of a self defined by contextual membership, but it adds a detail: the defining context is one substantially arranged by language exchanges between those who create the context. The consequences for a study of private lives and public structures are these: in looking at any event occurring within an individual, such as a static mental image, a memory, or a dream, one should be primarily interested in the *communication about* that event and only secondarily in the event itself. If that priority is obscured, then one has overlooked what is novel about a general systems view of behavior—namely, that it keeps one oriented to issues of contemporaneous information and the public transactional structures thereby created, rather than to the private, unobservable events of private life. As general systems theory—and its clinical derivative, structural family therapy—gives serious attention to the place of language in shaping public and private experience, then the task of integrating individual experience with observable family process may become easier.

THE STRUCTURAL APPROACH AND CLINICAL PRACTICE

The struggle to integrate psychodynamic with systemic theories will undoubtedly continue, in part because neither theory does enough justice to the preferred data of the other and in part because most people are uncomfortable with a pluralistic view of reality, preferring instead at least the belief in, if not the actual evidence for, a unified theory of behavior. Aside from these lofty concerns, the working clinician has more pragmatic and immediate final questions about structural family therapy. They mainly are questions about the limits and uses of this approach in daily practice.

The Limits of Structural Family Therapy

One of the major limits of this approach has already been discussed at length in the preceding section: the failure to move beyond a simply theoretical integration of the individual into the system and to achieve a truly detailed, clinically useful account as to how that happens. There are other problems, however. In the realm of everyday practice, two are often apparent, particularly for the beginning therapist.

First, structural therapists move relatively quickly in their efforts to restructure the family. There are a limited number of standardized moves available to do this. When these plays have been made, therapists using structural techniques may feel that the repertoire is exhausted and that they do not now know where to go next. Put simply, one may know how to get people to switch chairs, but how is the conversation then continued? Naturally, this is a limitation for beginning therapists who are so attentive to the mastery of the classic moves that they may be ill prepared to nuture the finer details of change. But even with experienced therapists, there seems to be a limited number of therapeutic moves within the structural model. A counterargument is that this limit is precisely the power of a structural viewpont—that simple, basic elements of family structure must be repetitively addressed before more complex content issues may be addressed. Perhaps that is so, but beginning structural therapists often find themselves suddenly without new moves to make and feel stuck in the repetition of the classic moves.

Second, the emphasis on a therapist as leader may eventuate in a rather authoritarian stance. There is a critical difference between an active therapist and an authoritarian one. Activity is encouraged, for the therapist must be leader and director as well as observer and follower of the family's own cues for change. But where progress is slow or when the classic moves have failed to produce change, one often sees therapists substitute irrational authority for leadership. This authority may even become a kind of enactment of the therapist's own frustration and an effort to conceal inept therapeutic planning. If confusion in the analytic situation is covered by even more silence on the analyst's part than is usual, then in most family therapy cases confusion is covered by even more activity on the part of the therapist. Activity and authoritarianism become blended in a stance that is not helpful to the family.

Additional limits of the clinical use of structural family therapy involve some confusion over the implicit behaviorism of the theory and an ambivalent stance toward interpretation. As for the role of behavior theory, structural family therapy makes no systematic or open use of traditional behaviorism, yet some implicit, though ill-formed notion of behavior modification is apparent in many of the clinical techniques. Ideas of reinforcement and extinction, of contingent reward, and of practice are clearly present in some of the tasks given by structural therapists. Yet these ideas are not explicitly outlined or developed. In a similar way, this usefulness of interpretation is dealt with in a mixed fashion. Although, as noted earlier, Minuchin advocated giving families descriptions of their process in an effort to alter their sense of collective reality, there is yet some reluctance to teach beginning therapists the exact referents of such description. Is "description" an ordering of facts that lie as close to observed reality as possible? Or can it hint at processes only inferred by the family? If the latter, perhaps descriptions of process are really much like traditional interpretations of hidden forces and feelings. Not too surprisingly, structural family therapy, in its efforts to differentiate itself sharply from the older analytic paradigm, expressly avoided interventions that looked like traditional interpretative techniques. Yet some form of explanation or description of process proved irresistible, perhaps, in a simple way, because people like to construct reasons about why things happen. At any rate, structural family therapy remains limited and unclear in its commitment to interpretation as an intervention strategy. People will talk, therapists most of all, and so some standard for the levels of description must be developed if beginning therapists are to comment clearly about the structures they observe.

The Uses of Structural Family Therapy

Because of the widely known *Families of the Slums* (Minuchin, Montalvo, Guerney, Rosman, & Schumer, 1967), the initial clinical application of structural therapy was to poor and disorganized families. A continued effort to confine this approach to the poor was a subtly discriminatory signal of resistance to the full potential of the therapy. Naturally, opponents argued, the poor, often characterized as creatures of action and impulse, needed "structuring" before they could attend to the deeper issues of psychological content. Since structural family therapy was itself active, even directive, it seemed ideal for a client population whose most visible qualities were the underorganization of family routines and transactional disengagements from each other. From such a perspective, structural family therapy could be viewed as a helpful adjunct to the traditional, psychodynamically oriented psychotherapies. Clinicians using the structural approach, however, knew that its usefulness was much wider; it was not a therapeutic technique designed for some limited clinical population, but a *theory* of change capable of application to many varieties of human disturbance. This point became dramatically apparent in Minuchin's work with anorectic children (Minuchin et al., 1978), most of whom came from white, middle- and upper-middle-class families. The success in treating these children, as well as children with other psychosomatic illnesses, demonstrated the efficacy of this therapy with problems traditionally treated only through a psychodynamic approach.

Errors of overestimation also occurred. There were problems of overinclusion—a sense that every disturbance would yield to the structural approach. As with all new ideologies, the initial struggle for recognition was followed by an insistence that structural therapy be used everywhere. In some quarters, this rather grand view still prevails. Aponte and Van Deusen (1981), for example, have claimed that structural family therapy is virtually without limits in its clinical applicability. More generally, however, structuralists have now become discriminating in their use of this approach and consequently are able to be more clear than they originally were about its usefulness. For example, the structural model is most powerful when applied to at least a two-generational family arrangement in which subgroups of parents and children can be examined in their exchanges with one another and with the outside world. Structural therapy has a great deal of influence over a clinician's view of how these subgroups are functioning and how they might change. The critical notions of interface transactions, hierarchies, alliances, and boundary are all extremely useful when one examines the internal workings of a two- or three-generational family system. On the other side, structural therapy has no particular purchase on a couple's system alone, except that the interventions routinely relate the couple's behavior to adjacent subsystems. Most couples therapy done by structuralists lacks the distinguishing marks of a basic systems theory model and closely resembles many other styles of couple psychotherapy. The single exception is an effort to recast a couple's behavior in terms of circular causality. (See the useful article by Stanton & Todd, 1979.)

Throughout the last two decades, structural family therapy has made its greatest mark in work with children, adolescents, and young adults still living at home. Aponte and Van Deusen's excellent review of structural family therapy has summarized some of the current uses of this approach. In reporting on 20 separate studies, the authors discussed work with four types of families: low socioeconomic status families, psychosomatic families, alcoholic families, and addict families. They were careful to note the substantial research difficulties created by the lack of comparable data—different studies used different study variables, different assessment methods, and so forth. In short, the research on structural family therapy outcome has suffered the fate of most psychotherapy outcome research. It has sometimes been banal, as when addict families have been described as ones with an active coalition between the mother and the son, while the father was disengaged, a description failing to discriminate between these families and dozens of other symptomatic types. Other research has produced results that have failed to distinguish it from any other therapeutic approach; for example, structural family therapy has done best with middle- and upper-class families with psychosomatic disorders and has been less effective with the poor. Nor has structural family therapy been explicitly combined with other types of therapeutic interventions. Moreover, only minimal research has been done on any of the specific techniques associated with structural family therapy. Studies of crisis induction have been an exception, and there has been some evidence that this has been an effective intervention technique. In trying to synthesize the various research findings, Aponte and Van Deusen were forced to note that, with regard to all categories of patient families, there were few uniform trends and that most summary statements were quite worthless. Take, for example, their statement that "Dysfunctional behaviors can lean toward either of two extremes. Communication may be dense or sparse, evenly distributed or skewed across family members; leadership may be authoritarian or anarchic, controlling or passive; affect may be blatantly protective or aggressive . . ." (p. 348). And so on. Despite such a disheartening welter of data and summaries, Aponte and Van Deusen nonetheless managed to offer some clear advantages of the structural approach.

They pointed out that there has been consistent evidence of dramatic improvement in both the symptomatic and psychosocial aspects of families with psychosomatic problems. Structural family therapy has been used with astounding success in the treatment of children with diabetic disorders, anorexia, asthma, and chronic pain problems. Minuchin's work with these psychosomatic families has constituted a persuasive application of structural techniques. The rate of improvement among these families was substantially better than previously achieved with other therapeutic efforts. The evidence on alcoholic and addict families has been less clear, however. Stanton and Todd (1979) reported significant reduction of addiction symptoms, although there was no corresponding improvement in psychosocial functioning. Overall, Aponte and Van Deusen attempted a summary of the 201 families included in those 20 studies and concluded that approximately 73 percent of these cases were effectively helped when treated by structural methods. The effectiveness varied from study to study, ranging between 50 to 100 percent.

The research on the efficacy of structural family therapy has suffered all the faults of most research on psychotherapy effectiveness. The usefulness of the technique has continued to be demonstrated by individual clinicians and not by the inconclusive statistics of poorly designed studies. The pessimism registered here is not about structural family therapy, but about the capacity of traditional behavioral science research to order its inquiries or operationalize its terms in a manner that has any meaningful relationship to clinical reality. Elegantly designed studies have usually been done at the expense of relevance, while research of any possible clinical substance has generally fallen far short of high marks for methodology. Replications have been few, and there has been little pressure to establish a continuity of terms or procedures that would bring one's present study into line with previous research efforts. Since there must be continuing efforts to assess the usefulness of structural family therapy, future researchers may avoid some of these design problems by avoiding large sample studies and turning instead to the single case approach. This has been very successfully used in the statistical evaluation of behavior therapy (Kratochwill, 1978; Hersen & Barlow, 1976) and could be applied to cases treated through family therapy.

Although anecdotes do not a science make, the advantages of structural family therapy, like those of other therapies, will continue to be argued from the viewpoint of clinical example. From that vantage point, many therapists, especially those who work with children and adolescents, feel that the perspectives and techniques of structural family therapy offer options for change never apparent in the more traditional child guidance model of therapy. To understand the context of a child's symptom is to grasp the ways in which that behavior is reinforced and hence resistant to the best efforts of individual child therapy. The uses of structural family therapy are most clearly demonstrated around issues with children, although proponents of the approach would argue its merits for a great variety of presenting problems. Clearly, structural family therapy can be overinclusive in its claims. Nonetheless, it affords a perspective on symptomatic behavior that frequently allows the therapist to move relatively quickly and effectively in efforts to change behavior.

THE STRUCTURAL ADVANTAGE

The achievement of Minuchin and his colleagues has been to distill from the intricate complexities of general systems theory a concise compendium of clinical strategies that offers the family therapist leverage for change. More than other theories of family therapy, structural family therapy achieves a fidelity to the organismic paradigm described through general systems theory. But while general systems theory is broad enough in its design to encompass many subordinate levels of human experience, structural family therapy, as a *theory,* has not led to new theoretical horizons. There really has been no "cutting edge" of the theory, no scurry of theorists to revise or expand its basic premises. When such explanation has been promoted as, for example, by Aponte and Van Deusen, who have claimed structural family therapy to be nearly universal in its inclusiveness, then, as Gurman (1981) has pointed out, the theory has become untestable and its techniques so diverse that knowledge as to which are critically helpful and which are not has been defied. What one may expect to see instead of theoretical expansions is a proliferation of studies applying the techniques of structural family therapy to different client groups. As a theory of family life, the structural viewpoint does well enough in translating some aspects of general systems theory into clinical strategies;

it need not be a grand theory of universal happenings. In fact, properly viewed, the structural theory is rather nicely proportioned to the techniques derived from it: the theory is neither too large to obscure the clinical strategies, nor is it too small to offer credible justifications for the use of these strategies. The structural approach provides a good enough theory for a good enough try at changing people.

In this matter of helping people change, the structural advantage is considerable. It teaches a therapist the beauty of position, of a place in the system from which one may grow or stagnate. Structural family therapy is preeminently a series of techniques for rearranging the parts of a living system so that adaptive growth and differentiation occur in accordance with the life-cycle demands of the surrounding culture as well as the internal agendas of the family itself. The attention to systems position is a distinctive advantage of the structural perspective. It alerts the therapist to the primacy of place and process, thereby helping one escape the often bewildering array of content issues brought by the family. No matter the sophistication or accuracy of one's attention to psychological nuance, if the perception of underlying structure falters, then all good and wise interpretations and interventions will also fail. This is the fundamental lesson of structural family therapy and one that, once learned, offers the therapist clear strategic advantages. When the alliances and hierarchies of a family are in harmony both with the family's own design for life and with the normative requirements of the larger culture, then experiences of contact and caring may unfold with benefit to all. Individual diversities and family unities thrive and endure when the structures of life are clearly seen. Eventually to see these structures is to move deeply beyond the protective coloring of everyday manners and to glimpse a totality remarkable in design and in action. The structural vision offers the therapist new avenues into the complex crossroads of family life. Those routes make for wonderful travels.

GLOSSARY

accommodation Describes one way of joining a family in order to form a therapeutic unit. In accommodation, the therapist knowingly conforms to the transactional structures and communicational rules of the family system. See also *induction* as unknowing accommodation.

alliance Designates a positive affinity between two units of the system. This is the popular usage of the term, not a formal definition. An alliance is potentially neutral, though it carries with it an inherent capability to become assertively directed against a third party. When alliances stand in opposition to another part of the system, then one may speak of coalitions. See also *coalition.*

behavior-exchange sequence Refers to the transformation of psychological content into observable behaviors that are exchanged across subsystem boundaries. Content events occurring totally within a subsystem are usually unobservable and can only be inferred. When, however, the content results in interpersonal contact, then behaviors occur in sequence, among subsystems, and these exchanges may be observed.

boundary A boundary is a metaphor that stands for particular, regularly occurring transactions between subsystems. These transactions regulate the amount and kind of information and the energy that flows from one subsystem to another. This variation in flow is symbolized by speaking of the relative "closedness" or "openness" of a boundary. Boundaries may also assume tangible form, as in houses with heavily curtained windows and double-locked doors or in homes where there are no doors between any of the rooms and where no physical structures designate separate subsystem functions. A boundary is also a metaphorical statement about accessibility to a subsystem.

change From a systems viewpoint, change may occur when pressures within the family group result in a shift to a different systems design and a new homeostatic relationship, or when forces from outside the family, such as a therapist, create a crisis and hence pressure for different behaviors. The process of change may not be a continuous, stepwise event, but instead may occur in discontinuous, sudden leaps to new organizational patterns. Both part and whole must change in some conjunction with each other, though not always simultaneously.

coalition Designates an arrangement, generally involving several or many family members, in which there is a combative, exclusionary, or scapegoating stance toward a third party. Coalitions popularly refer to arrangements among more than two people. See also *alliance.*

complexity Used here to designate a desirable progression within living systems from a relatively undifferentiated arrangement of functions to a more multifaceted arrangement, whereby multiple adaptive activities are carried out simultaneously. The more complex a system's development, the less likely it is to become seriously dysfunctional in the face of individual symptomatology. Conversely, the less complex the development, the more rigid the system in dealing with stress.

constancy loops Feedback loops that promote homeostasis can be referred to as constancy loops, that is, feedback processes that ensure conformance to the dominant parameters of the system's overall design for living. See also *deviation-countering feedback loops.*

content In family systems theory, content refers to the particular themes and concretized attributes of life that, joined together through time, give thematic meaning to the daily activities of a family and its members. Content refers to the psychological phenomena that are the substance of systems concepts such as information and energy. See also *information* and *energy.*

context Refers to the properties of a living system and to the physical, social, and psychological environment in which the system is itself embedded. With regard to any particular system or subsystem, a context exists (1) when there is a collectivity of parts that surround and stand in an adjacent and dynamic relationship to that focal part, and (2) when this collectivity of surrounding parts conforms to the operating principles of general systems theory.

crisis Designates a period in family process when the customary ways of responding to stimuli are blocked, thereby creating an experience of collective trial-and-error behavioral exchanges and instances of individual upset. A crisis period is viewed by structuralists as a necessary prelude to change, since it moves the family away from states of stagnant homeostasis. Minuchin (Minuchin & Barcai, 1969) contrasts crisis with "emergency," which refers to the chronic recurrence of some symptom and to the family's efforts to manage it with familiar strategies.

deviation-amplifying feedback loops This is another designation for variety loops. When some deviation from the family's baseline design for living is signaled, then this deviation is amplified by supportive moves from other parts of the system. Deviation-amplifying feedback loops promote growth and change within the system. An overabundance of such feedback activity may result in a crisis and temporary breakdown of the system, thereby setting the stage for necessary change. See also *variety loops.*

deviation-countering feedback loops This is another designation for constancy loops. When some deviation from the family's baseline design for living is signaled, then this deviation is countered, that is, corrected by countervailing moves from other parts of the system. Deviation-countering loops promote homeostasis. An overabundance of such feedback activity may result in pathological stagnation of the system. See also *constancy loops.*

disengaged Refers to families with depleted sensitivity to its individual members and low systems resonance. Interpersonal distances are too great, and subsystem boundaries are too rigid. Individual behaviors are seldom noticed or have little potential to activate the system. See also *enmeshed.*

energy Refers to the emotional force, repetition, and duration of any particular communication signal, whether occurring totally within the boundaries of a single subsystem or occurring across boundaries. Energy refers to the force and rate of exchange evident around the transmission of these signals.

enmeshed Refers to families in which there is extreme sensitivity among the individual members to each other and to their primary subsystem. Even small behaviors reverberate quickly and with increasing magnitude throughout the entire system. There is little interpersonal distance and considerable blurring of boundaries. See also *disengaged.*

feedback loop A cybernetic term referring to communicational processes that circle across subsystem boundaries and back again, signaling to the members of that unit their degree of conformity to or difference from some overall purpose of the system. Emphasis is on the circularity of this constantly self-correcting process.

hierarchy As used in general systems theory, this refers to a rule of ordering such that some elements of a system are subordinate to other elements. All living systems arrange themselves into hierarchic orders in order to promote the differentiation of system parts and the increasing complexity of the whole. Hierarchical ordering makes it possible for any particular element to be simultaneously a whole encompassing subordinate parts and a part of a superordinate whole.

holon Describes the component parts of a system so that each may be simultaneously considered a whole in its own right, but also a part of some larger entity in which it is embedded. For example, one may be an individual and at the same time a member of the marital unit. A holon strives for self-preservation as a whole, but also contributes integrative energy as a part. See *subsystem.*

homeostasis The relatively steady state a system achieves for substantial periods of time. Homeostasis is a dynamic equilibrium during which time the system functions without undue stress on its component parts. It represents an idealized period of balance, often contrasted to periods of crisis or disequilibrium. See also *constancy loops.*

index patient A term used to designate the individual family member whose behavior is labeled as problematic. This use of an individual label may lead to an incorrect labeling of the entire family, as in referring to "schizophrenic families" or "drug addiction families."

induction The unknowing compliance of the therapist to the transactional structures and communicational rules of the family system. Induction is unwitting accommodation to the family patterns and occurs frequently in the initial phases of therapy.

information A term used in general systems theory to designate the signals, verbal and nonverbal, used by a system or its subsystems to tell the participants how well they are conforming to or differing from the established goals and purposes of the family group. The conveyance of such information is vital in helping a family group respond adaptively and healthily to the changing requirements of its environment. See also *system design.*

interface Designates a point in transactional experience when the behavioral operations of one system extend into contact with those of another system. At that moment, the two systems are adjacent to each other and are attempting to influence the behavioral strategies of the other system. Therapists who observe and attempt to change the behavioral sequences exchanged between the adjacent systems may be said to be "working at the interface."

morphogenesis A general systems theory term that designates a change in the structural arrangement of a system's parts such that the total system acquires new adaptive strategies and possibilities. See also *change.*

morphostasis A general systems theory term that designates a constancy in the structural arrangement of a system's parts such that the total system continues its current pattern of adaptive strategies and possibilities. See *homeostasis.*

organismic paradigm A conceptual model for explaining behavior. It is derived from general systems theory and emphasizes the reality of circular causality rather than that of linear causality.

pathology In systems terms, pathology refers to (1) increased rigidity of transactional behavior, (2) persistently closed boundaries between subsystems, and (3) continued avoidance of alternative behaviors. More abstractly, a pathological family is one stuck in chronic states of homeostasis, one that allows no crisis to move it to new and more adaptive states of functioning.

process Refers to a discrete, time-limited sequence of behaviors that make up any particular transactions among the system components. A process consists of linked behavioral exchanges. In contrast to structure, which has the qualities of repetition and duration, processes are single behavioral occurrences of short duration. See also *structure.*

redefinition In clinical theory, redefinition is a shift of perspective from the individual patient to the family system; as such, it allows for a new meaning of the individual symptom. In clinical practice, the shift may be shared with the family as a *reframing* of the presenting problem so that individual behaviors are now seen as linked to a meaningful family pattern.

reframing See *redefinition.*

rule A persistent patterning in family interactions may assume the status of a rule. Some rules are intentionally announced and followed, as in a family that describes itself as "close-knit and without fighting." The more important rules, however, are often outside of the family's awareness and are composed of the repetitive behaviors that make up the routines of daily family life. These behaviors are rule-governed insofar as deviation from the routine evokes awareness that something new has occurred.

sequence Refers to a repeating cycle of linked behaviors. A sequence is often analyzed and recognized as a linear event, inasmuch as each step in the cycle is followed by another. But since the final step in the progression is always the occasion to return to the beginning of the cycle, a sequence in fact describes a circular and repetitive unfolding of linked behaviors.

staging Refers to the division of a therapeutic intervention into separate and self-contained units, which are themselves arranged in some sort of logical progression. An entire treatment plan may be staged, as when the therapist begins with the entire family and then moves to progressively smaller family units. Or a single intervention may be staged, as when a therapist asks some central family members first to sit next to each other and then to begin a dialogue without interruption from other family members.

structural therapy Used here as a short form for structural family therapy.

structure Refers to the interactional patterns that arrange or organize a family's component subsystems into somewhat constant relationships. These constant relationships are enduring through time, but less so than the continuous activity of the superordinate, total system. That is, the system, as an entity, continues through the family's entire lifetime while various structures, or organizational arrangements of the components, will shift and change from time to time. Structures are seen in the relatively stable subsystems, alliances, and hierarchies that characterize a family's organizational map. Structures may also be thought of as slow processes of long duration. See also *process.*

subsystem A subsystem is one element of the total system. It may comprise a single person or several persons joined together by common membership criteria, such as age, sex, or shared purpose. These subsystems exist in a state of dynamic interchange with contiguous subsystems. They are organized around the performance of functions crucial to their own well-being and to that of the total system. See also *subunit* and *holon.*

subunit See *subsystem* and *holon.*

symptom Refers to behaviors that signal dysfunction both in individuals and in the whole family. While both psychodynamic and systems theory argue that a symptom indicates wider circles of pathology, the family viewpoint also argues that the symptom be a focus of intervention as well as of treatment of the interpersonal context in which it is embedded.

system A system is a set of units, themselves organized into an interdependent whole, which, as a living phenomenon, is something different from and greater than a simple adding-up of the parts. A system contains a set of interrelating elements and, as a totality, shows a capacity for performance, especially in regard to adaptation to the surrounding environment. A system has a capacity to endure over time, although elements of the system and the system itself will be undergoing periods of transformation, as dictated by pressures for change that come from both inside and outside the system.

system design The design of a system refers to the established, often idealized purposes and goals of family life and to the style in which these goals are to be reached. This design governs, on an intentional level, much of the informational signals that are transmitted throughout all the subsystems of the family.

therapeutic unit In family systems therapy, the unit within which healing occurs is composed of the family plus the therapist. This is in contrast to other therapies, which attempt to place the therapist in a disengaged and neutral position and hence outside the boundaries of the client unit.

tracking A procedure whereby the therapist helps the family elaborate the details of behavioral routines so that a coherent picture emerges of any particular complaint. To track the content of family life is to promote this complete elaboration. Tracking also involves a therapeutic possibility—namely, that the extended inquiry into facets of family life will subtly guide the family to a new and expanded version of reality, which takes the focus off of the index patient.

triangles A favorite structural unit used by systems theorists in describing family functioning. A triangle consists of three subsystems joined together by mutual interests, complementary responsibilities (as with parents and a child), or competitive entanglements. Triangles are viewed by structuralists as inherently unstable, tending periodically to resolve themselves into arrangements of two against one. There is nothing pathological about this tendency as long as membership in the "in-group" shifts from time to time.

triangulation Refers to a psychological process, involving traditional, psychodynamic operations whereby a unit of two stabilizes itself and gives meaning to its activity through common reference to a third unit. This is apparent, for example, in marital units in which persistent harmony depends on equally persistent anger or benevolent concern toward a child (the third unit). The meaning of membership in a subsystem may be best experienced through shared reference to a third unit that lies outside the boundaries of the subsystem.

variety loops Feedback loops that promote fluctuation and change in systems operations. These feedback processes ensure that a living system will respond adaptively to the pressures for growth that come from both outside and inside the system. See also *deviation-amplifying feedback loops.*

REFERENCES

Aponte, H., & Hoffman, L. The open door: A structural approach to a family with an anorectic child. *Family Process,* 1973, *12,* 1–44.

Aponte, H., & Van Deusen, J. Structural family therapy. In A. Gurman (Ed.), *Handbook of family therapy.* New York: Brunner/Mazel, 1981.

Bateson, G. *Steps to an ecology of mind.* New York: Ballantine, 1972.

Bateson, G., Jackson, D., Haley, J., & Weakland, J. Toward a theory of schizophrenia. *Behavioral Science,* 1956, *1.*

Beavers, W.R. *Psychotherapy and growth.* New York: Brunner/Mazel, 1977.

Boszormenyi-Nagy, I., & Spark, G. *Invisible Loyalties.* New York: Harper & Row, 1973.

Bowen, M. *Family Therapy in Clinical Practice.* New York: Jason Aronson, 1978.

Buckley, W. *Sociology and modern system theory.* Englewood Cliffs, N.J.: Prentice-Hall, 1967.

Buckley, W. (Ed.). *Modern systems research for the behavioral scientist.* Chicago: Aldine, 1968.

Caille, P. The Evaluation Phase of Systemic Family Therapy. *Journal of Marital and Family Therapy,* Jan. 1979, 29–39.

Caplow, T. *Two against one: Coalitions in triads.* Englewood Cliffs, N.J.: Prentice-Hall, 1968.

Dell, P. Beyond homeostasis: Toward a concept of coherence. *Family Process,* 1982, *21,* 21–41.

Dell, P., & Goolishian, H. Order through fluctuation. Paper presented at the Annual Scientific Meeting of the A.K. Rice Institute, Houston, Texas, 1979.

Dell, P., & Goolishian, H. Order through fluctuation: An evolutionary epistemology for human systems. *Australian Journal of Family Therapy,* 1981, *2,* 175–184.

Glansdorff, P., & Prigogine, I. *Thermodynamic theory of structure, stability, and fluctuations.* New York: John Wiley & Sons, 1971.

Gurman, A. (Ed.). *Handbook of family therapy.* New York: Brunner/Mazel, 1981.

Haley, J. *Strategies of psychotherapy*. New York: Grune & Stratton, 1963.

Haley, J. *Problem-solving therapy*. San Francisco: Jossey-Bass, 1976.

Haley, J. *Leaving home*. New York: McGraw-Hill, 1980.

Hersen, M., & Barlow, D. *Single case experimental designs: Strategies for studying behavior change*. New York: Pergamon Press, 1976.

Hoffman, L. Deviation-amplifying processes in natural groups. In J. Haley (Ed.), *Changing families*. New York: Grune & Stratton, 1971.

Hoffman, L. The family life cycle and discontinuous change. In E. Carter & M. Orfanides (Eds.), *The family life cycle*. New York: Gardner Press, 1980.

Hoffman, L. *Foundations of family therapy*. New York: Basic Books, 1981.

Kantor, D. Critical identity image: A concept linking individual, couple, and family development. In J. Pearce & L. J. Friedman (Eds.), *Family therapy: Combining psychodynamic and family systems approaches*. New York: Grune & Stratton, 1980.

Kantor, D., & Lehr, W. *Inside the family*. San Francisco: Jossey-Bass, 1975.

Koestler, A. *Janus: A summing up*. New York: Vintage Books, 1979.

Kratochwill, T.R. (Ed.). *Single subject research: Strategies for evaluating change*. New York: Academic Press, 1978.

Madanes, Cloé. Protection, paradox, and pretending. *Family Process*, 1980, *19*, 73–85.

Maruyama, M. The second cybernetics: Deviation-amplifying mutual causal process. In W. Buckley (Ed.), *Modern systems research for the behavioral scientist*. Chicago: Aldine, 1968.

Miller, J. Living systems: Basic concepts. *Behavioral Science*, 1965, *10*(3), 193–237.

Minuchin, S. *Families and family therapy*. Cambridge, Massachusetts: Harvard University Press, 1974.

Minuchin, S. & Barcai, A. Therapeutically induced family crisis. In J. Masserman (Ed.), *Science and psychoanalysis*, Vol. 14. New York: Grune & Stratton, 1969, 199–205.

Minuchin, S., & Fishman, H.C. *Family therapy techniques*. Cambridge, Massachusetts: Harvard University Press, 1981.

Minuchin, S., Montalvo, B., Guerney, G., Rosman, B., & Schumer, F. *Families of the slums*. New York: Basic Books, 1967.

Minuchin, S., Roseman, B.L., & Baker, L. *Psychosomatic families: Anorexia nervosa in context*. Cambridge, Massachusetts: Harvard University Press, 1978.

Montalvo, B. "A family with a little fire" (videotape). Philadephia Child Guidance Cinic.

Palazzoli, M.S., Cecchin, G., Prata, G., & Boscolo, L. *Paradox and counterparadox*. New York: Jason Aronson, 1978.

Papp, P. The use of Paradox. In S. Minuchin & C. Fishman (Eds.), *Family Therapy Techniques*. Cambridge, Massachusetts: Harvard University Press 1981.

Rabkin, R. *Inner and outer space*. New York: W. W. Norton, 1970.

Sanders, F. *Individual and family therapy: Toward an integration*. New York: Jason Aronson, 1979.

Schafer, R. *Language and insight.* New Haven: Yale University Press, 1978.

Slipp, S. Interactions between the interpersonal in families and individual intrapsychic dynamics. In J. Pearce & L.J. Friedman (Eds.), *Family Therapy: Combining psychodynamic and family systems approaches.* New York: Grune & Stratton, 1980.

Stanton, M. D., & Todd, T. C. Structural family therapy with drug addicts. In E. Kaufman & P. Kaufman (Eds.), *The family therapy of drug and alcohol abuse.* New York: Gardner Press, 1979.

Umbarger, C., & Bernstein, A. "Getting out: Therapeutic rule breaking in an enmeshed system" (videotape). Family Institute of Cambridge, Cambridge, Massachusetts, 1979.

Umbarger, C., & Hare, R. A structural approach to patient and therapist disengagement from a schizophrenic family. *American Journal of Psychotherapy,* 1973, *27,* 274–284.

Umbarger, C., & White, S. Redefining the problem: Individual symptom and family system. *International Journal of Family Counseling,* 1978, *6*(2), 33–47.

von Bertalanffy, L. *General system theory* (rev. ed.). New York: George Braziller, 1968.

Walrond-Skinner, S. *Family therapy: The treatment of natural systems.* London: Routledge & Kegan Paul, 1976.

INDEX

Page numbers in *italics* refer to figures; page numbers followed by t refer to tables.